AF540123

Dictionary of Food and Nutrition

DICTIONARY OF FOOD AND NUTRITION

Bhavana Sabarwal

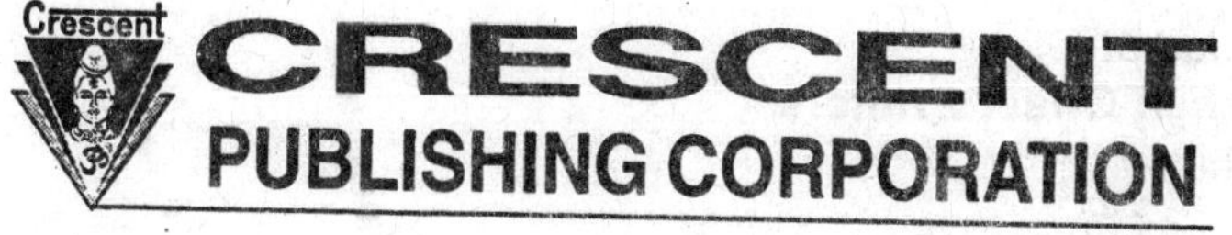

[The responsibility for the facts stated, conclusions reached and plagiarism, if any, in this book is entirely that of the Author. And the Publisher bears no responsibility for them, whatsoever.]

Dictionary of Food and Nutrition

First Published : 2012

ISBN 978-81-8342-226-0

Published by :

CRESCENT PUBLISHING CORPORATION
4819/24, Mathur Lane,
Ansari Road, Darya Ganj,
New Delhi - 110002
Mob. : 9711991838
Fax : 91- 011- 23257835
e-mail : crescentbook@gmail.com

Printed at :
Roshan Offset Printers
Delhi

PREFACE

This Compact *Dictionary of Food and Nutrition* is a valuable and reliable. In this Dictionary presentation of words to be used by the school and college students, teachers, common users, translators and researchers in the field. This Dictionary has been compiled and prepared after consulting various dictionaries available in the market. We have tried our best to present before you the updated forms of words being used in day to day life. The modern approach to information technology has been taken into account in the presentation of different types of words frequently used in modern perspective. It is clear from the pronunciation of word and syllable, which has the common usage.

The work will be revised and updated from time to time to keep it continuously useful and interesting. This Dictionary caters the needs of every user in his daily reading and writing. All efforts have been made to present accurate and adequate selection of words having common approach to all the sundry specially school-goers. Common and important vocabulary of daily used have been provided in composite forms so as to make them easily available at one place systematically.

Bhavana Sabarwal

A

Absorption. The active taking up of digested food nutrients through the villi of the small intestine into blood capillaries. Absorption is also a more general process in which substances, electromagnetic radiation or energy are taken up by other substances.

Accelerated Freeze Drying. Freeze drying carried out in conditions which speed up the *process, e.g.* with heating.

Acceptance-preference Test. Sensory analysis in which the Acceptability or desirability of the food product is determined. These kinds of test are commonly used with consumers.

Acesulfames. Also called acesulphames. Class of artificial, non- nutritive sweeteners from oxathiazinone. The potassium salt, called acesulfam-K, has been 200 times as sweet as sucrose; not metabolised and excreted unchanged; good self life.

Acetate, Active. Refers to the forms in which the acetyl radical, CH_2CO–, gets transferred from one compound to another, as the acetyl-coenzyme A complex (coenzyme A). The metabolism both of glucose and of fats involves the formation of active acetate.

Acetate Replacement Factor. Lipoic acid.

Acetic Acid. One of the simplest organic acids– CH_3 COOH, which is obtained by fermentation of ethyl alcohol (secondary fermentation) and formed in some fermented foods together with lactic acid, both of which serve to preserve such foods—i.e. the process of pickling. It is also added to foods and sauces to preserve them.

Acetobacter. Genus of bacteria of family Bacteriaceae. It oxidises alcohol to acetic acid. Acetobacter pasteurianus (also termed as Mycoderma aceti and Becterium aceti or pasteurianum) is used in the manufacture of vinegar. They grow in film on beer wort, pickle brine and fruit juices.

Acetoglycerides. They differ from the triglycerides in that either one or two of the long-chain fatty acids attached to the glycerol molecule get replaced by acetic acid. There are three types: diacetotriglycerides (e.g. monoacetomonostearin); monoacetotriglycerides (e.g. diacetodistearin); and monoacetodiglycerides (e.g. monoacetomonostearin), in which one hydroxyl group of the glycerol is free. Also termed as partial glyceride esters.

They are non-greasy and are having lower melting points than the corresponding triglycerides, and find use in shortenings and spreads, as films for coating foods, and as plasticisers for hard fats.

Acetoin. Acetyl methyl carbinol $CH_3COCHOHCH_3$. It is the precursor of diacetyl, butter flavour. It is produced by bacteria during butter ripening and by the yeast during fermentation.

Acetone Bodies. See Ketone bodies.

Acetylcholine. Acetyl derivative of Choline which gets liberated at certain nerve endings (cholinergic nerves) to stimulate the muscle.

ACH Index. Arm, chest, hip index. The arm girth, chest diameter and hip width. It finds use as a method of assessing the state of nutrition.

Achlorhydria. Refers to the deficiency of hydrochloric acid in the gastric secretion.

Achrodextrin. A product which is formed during the enzymic break-down of starch to maltose; it is a dextrin that does not give colour with iodine (hence achro).

Achromotrichia. Loss of hair pigment.

Acid (n). A compound which can lose protons i.e. hydrogen (H_4) ions and donate them to water forming H_3–O^+ ions acidic.

Acid-base Balance. Body fluids have been maintained just on the alkaline side of neutrality, pH *7.3-7.45,* by buffers in the blood and tissues. Buffers include proteins, and sodium and potassium phosphate and bicarbonate.

Acidic products of the body's metabolism get excreted in the urine in combination with bases like sodium and potassium. These bases are thereby lost to the body and the acid-base balance is maintained by replacing them from the diet.

Buffer materials in the blood and tissues are termed the alkaline reserve.

Acid Foods and Basic Foods. The term used for the residue of the metabolism of the food—the minerals sodium, potassium, magnesium and calcium are base-forming, and which of these predominates determines whether the food leaves an acid or basic residue. Meat, fish, eggs, cheese and cereals leave an acid or basic residue; milk, vegetables and some fruits leave an alkaline residue; fats and sugar contain no minerals and so are neutral foods.

Fruit juices are having acids and their sodium salts and have an acid taste, but the organic portion is completely oxidised and the residual sodium leaves an alkaline residue.

Acid Number. With reference to fats, this term refers to a measure of hydrolytic rancidity. It may be defined as milligrams of caustic potash required to neutralise the free fatty acids in 1g of the fat. The acid number, also known as the acid value, refers to an index of the efficiency of refining, during which process the free fatty acids are removed and the acid number falls to very low values. It is also an index of the deterioration in storage.

Acidophilus Therapy. Consumption of milk having a high concentration of viable Lactobacillus acidophilus (the milk itself being unfermented) as a treatment for constipation. The effect is said to be due to the implantation of these organisms in the intestine.

Acidosis. Refers to an increase in the ratio between acid and base in the blood plasma, or a reduction in its buffering power. Causes may be alteration in carbon dioxide excretion, metabolic overproduction of acid or excessive loss of base.

Acid Rebound. Term used in reference to the secretion of gastric acid to signify the increase in acidity of the stomach that results from the administration of alkalies. There-is conflicting evidence as to whether this really occurs.

Acid Value. See Acid number.

Ackee. Fruit of Blighia sapida which is common in West Indies. Unripe fruits have hypoglycin (α-amino-β-methylene cyclopropanylpropopionic acid-hypoglycin A, and its peptide- hypoglycin B) in quantities sufficient to reduce blood glucose levels and cause 'vomiting sickness', coma death.

Aconitine. Refers to toxic alkaloid of monkshood (Aconitum.) It slows the pulse and reduces blood pressure; fatal in small doses.

Acorn Sugar. Quercitol. It is extracted from acorns. It is pentahydroxycyclohexane.

ACP. Acid calcium phosphate.

Acraldehyde. See Acrolein.

Acrodynia. Speciphic type of dermatit is seen in animals that are fed on diet deficient in vitamin B_6.

Actin. A globular protein which takes part in the contraction of muscle through the formation of the thin filaments and their interaction with the thick filaments.

Activators. With reference to enzymes, these are substances that are able to increase the activity of the enzyme in a non-specific manner. Those substances that are part of the activating system, and are required before the enzyme can activate its substrate, are activators. Substances that are part of the reaction system but play no part in the activation of the substrate are coenzymes.

Many inorganic radicals are activators; thus salivary amylase requires the presence of chloride; others are potassium, calcium, magnesium, phosphate.

Active Oxygen Method. Refers to a method of measuring the stability of fats and oils by bubbling air through the heated material and following the formation of peroxides. Also known as the Swift stability test.

Active Site. The part of the enzyme molecule which interacts with the substrate and where the catalysis of the reaction takes place. The active site usually has a special shape so that the substrates can bond to it.

Actomyosin. A protein aggregate formed when actin and myosin interact during muscle contraction.

Addison's Disease. Refers to destruction of the cortex of the suprarenal glands. Its symptoms are low blood pressure, anaemia; muscular weakness, fall in metabolic rate. Treatment partly successful by taking sodium chloride, or by implantation of pellets of deoxycorticosterone acetate.

Additive. A substance added to food to aid processing preservation to improve flavour or colour, e.g., pigments lakes emulsifiers, flavouring, humectants, stabilizers, vitamins, minerals.

Adenosine. Combination of the base adenine with the sugar ribose.

Adenosine Diphosphate (ADP). Adenosine nucleotides.

Adenosine Monophosphate. See Adenylic acid.

Adenosine Nucleotides. Adenosine triphosphate (ATP) is having three phosphate moieties esterified to adenosine. Two of these gets associated with a high free energy of hydrolysis, and are also called 'high-energy' Phosphates; they are readily available for transfer to other compounds, and are a common method of energy transfer in reaction. In general, oxidative (energy- yielding) metabolism gives rise to the synthesis of ATP from ADP, while synthetic reactions, which require energy, involve the use of phosphate from ATP to yield ADP (adenosine diphosphate).

Cyclic AMP gets formed from ATP by the action of adenyl cyclase; the enzyme is frequently activated in cell membranes by hormones and neurotransmitters, and acts as a second messenger for a hormone; it is common allosteric effector of regularly enzymes.

Adenosine Triphosphate. See Adenosine nucleotides.

Addenylic Acid. Combination of the base adenine with the sugar ribose, and phosphoric acid. It is also known as adenosine monophosphoric acid. It is also known as adenosine monophosphate or AMP; of importance in muscle metabolism.

Adipose Tissue. Groups of cells that are able to store and mobilise fat; constitutes one-fifth to one-quarter of the total body mass— more in fat people. Composed of 82-88% fat, 2-2.6% protein and 10-14% water and has 8-9 kcal (34-38 KJ) per gram or 3600-4000 (15.1-16.8 MJ) per pound.

Adlay. Refers to tall grass. Coix lacharyma-jobi, Jobs's tears. It grows wild in parts of Africa and Asia. It is used as a cereal to take out rice supplies in countries in S.E. Pacific area. Same tribe as maize Tripsaceae. Analysis per 100 g: 14 g protein, 4 g fat, 4 mg Fe, 0.3 mg vitamin B_1, 0.2 mg vitamin B_2, 3 mg niacin, 360 kcal *(1.5 141).*

ADI. Acceptable daily intake: refers to chemical additives used in food processing.

Adipose Tissue. Tissues containing cells filled with lips stored in vacuoles. It is the growth of adipose tissue which causes obesity. However, adipose tissue is a normal part of every animal body and is necessary for storing lipids as a source of energy.

ADP. Adenosine diphosphate. The nucleotide which is formed from the hydrolysis of ATP. It contains two phosphate groups.

Adrenal Glands. Also called suprarenal glands. These are situated just above each kidney. Comprise the inner part, or medulla, which secretes adrenaline and noradrenaline (which see), and the outer cortex, which secretes steriod hormones.

Examples of steriod hormones are steroid sex hormones, corticosterone (affects carbohydrate metabolism and is anti-inflammatory) and aldosterone (controls excretion of salt and water through the kidneys).

Adrenaline. A hormone which gets secreted by the medullas of the adrenal glands; the first hormone to be discovered. It gets secreted under conditions of emotional stress, and causes an increase in blood pressure, blood sugar levels and metabolic rate, thus mobilising the body's reserves of energy.

It is also known as epinephrine, chemically hydroxy, dihydroxyphenyl-ethylmethylamine.

Adrenocorticotropic Hormone. A hormone which is extracted from the anterior part of the pituitary gland of animals and used in the treatment of rheumatoid arthritis. Acts by stimulating the adrenal gland to secrets corticosteroids.

Aequum. Refers to an amount of food which is necessary to maintain body weight under normal or specified conditions of activity (rarely used).

Aeration. The mixing of small air bubbles with a substance, for example with, fat or oil during the process of creaming.

Aerobes. Micro-organisms that need oxygen for growth. Obligate aerobes cannot survive in the absence of oxygen.

Aerosol. A colloid in which the disperse phase is a solid or a liquid and the continuous phase is a gas e.g. fog, mist.

Aesculin (Esculin). Dihydroxycoumarin glucoside found in the leaves and the bark of the chestnut tree, Aesculus hippocastanum. Has affect on Capillary fragility, which see.

AFD. Accelerated freeze-drying.

Aflatoxin. Refers to toxic metabolite of the mould Aspergillus Flavus. It was first identified as an outbreak of Turkey X disease in the UK in 1960 due to consumption of infected groundnuts; since found in a wide variety of nuts and cereals.

Aflatoxin B_1 has been both acutely toxic and carcinogen

in experimental animals, but human beings appear to be relatively resistant to the carcinogenic effect. When aflatoxin B_1 is consumed by dairy cows, a metabolite, aflatoxin M_1, is found in the milk and cheese.

Agar. Dried, purified stems of a seaweed, Gelidium algae, Gracilaria and other genera. It is partly soluble, and swells with water to form a gel it has a wide temperature range between gelling and melting points.

It finds use in soups, jellies, ice-cream, meat and fish pastes, in bacteriological media, for sizing silk, as adhesive and as a stabiliser for emulsions. Also called agar-agar, Macassar gum and vegetable gelatine.

Agar is a galactan, i.e. a complex of galactose units, but it is not digested by man.

Agene. Nitrogen trichloride. It was once used as bleaching and 'improving' agent for wheat flour in bread making but found to react with methionine to form methionine sulphoximine, which caused 'canine hysteria' and so was abandoned.

Ageusia. Lack or impairment of sensitivity to taste stimuli.

Agglomeration. Refers to production of a free-flowing, dust free power from substances such as dried milk powder and wheat flour. The process consists of moistening with droplets of water and drying in a stream of air; the agglomerates are readily wettable.

Aggregate. A gathering of molecules, Particles.

Aging.

1. Term applied to chemicals which are used to oxidise (age) wheat flour for bread making. Freshly milled flour produces a weaker and less resilient dough and less 'bold' loaf than flour which has been stored for some weeks or 'aged' chemically. Substances like ammonium persulphate, ascorbic acid, chlorin, sulphur dioxide, potassium bromate and cysteine are used as oxidising agents; nitrogen peroxide and benzoyl peroxide, to bleach the flour; chlorine dioxide (and at one time nitrogen trichloride-agene), to bleach the flour and 'improve' the dough. Regulations in countries control which of these

may be used.

2. In reference to wine aging. This terms refers to the development of a 'bouguet' and smooth, mellow flavour and the disappearance of harsh yeasty flavours by slow oxidation and the formation of esters.

Aglycon. Refers to the non-sugar part of a glucoside.

Agnellato. Envelop of pasta which has been stuffed with minced meat or vegetables; cut in half-moon shape, so differing form ravioli, which is cut in squares.

A/G Ratio. Albumin/globulin ratio.

Air Classification. Separation of fractions of powdered material in a current of air on the basis of size and composition of the particles. Particularly applied to fractionation of the endosperm of milled wheat flour; the smaller particles are richer on protein-fraction range from 3% to 25% protein.

Alanine. Refers to a non-essential amino acid, amino propionic acid. The alpha amino acid occurs in all proteins; there is also betaalanine (the amino group attached to the second carbon atom), which is part of the molecule of pantothenic acid, of carnosine and of anserine.

Albedo. White pith of the inner peel or citrus fruits. It is also known as the mesocarp; 20-60% of the whole fruit. It is having sugar, cellulose and pectins; used as a source of pectin for commercial manufacture.

Albumen. Oxford Dictionary spelling of albumin.

Albumin. A simple protein soluble in water and coagulated by heat, for example, lactalbumin in milk, ovalbumin in egg, and serum albumin in blood.

Albumin/globulin Ratio. Refers to ratio between the blood albumin and the globulins; in normal human serum, 1.82. Change in the A/G ratio is of diagnostic value.

Albumin Index. Refers to a measure of the quality of an egg. It is the ratio between the height of the albumin and the width when broken on to a flat surface. As the egg deteriorates, the albumin index gets decreased, i.e. the egg white spreads.

Albuminoids (scleroproteins). Fibrous proteins that are having supporting or protective function in animals (in plants cellulose fulfils this function) Three types:

1. Collagens in skin, tendons and bones, resistant to pepsin and trypsin, covered to water soluble gelatin by boiling with water,
2. Elastins in tendons and arteries, not coverted to gelatin;
3. Keratins, protein insoluble in dilute acids and alkalies, not attacked by any animal digestive enzymes, comprise horns, hoofs feathers, scales, nails.

Albumoses. Old name for proteoses.

Alcaptonuria. Refers to a rare inborn error of metabolism of the two amino acids phenylalanine and tyrosine. Their metabolism ceases at homogentisic acid, which gets excreted in the urine. Homogentistic acid oxidises to black melanoid pigments; hence, the urine of alcaptonurics slowly turns black. The defect appears to be harmless.

Alcohol. Generally it refers to ethyl alcohol or ethanol C_2H_5OH, although it is the second member of the series of alcohols of the general formula CnH_{2n+1} OH. It is obtained by yeast fermentation of sugars, and the basis of a large number of alcoholic beverages ranging from low alcohol beers containing 2% ethanol to spirits with 30%.

Alcohol, Denatured. Alcohol to which unpleasant materials are added to prevent in being drunk-e.g. methylated spirits contains 10% methyl alcohol, a blue dye and unpleasant smelling pyridine. Denatured alcohol finds use for industrial purposes and not subject to Excise Duty.

Alcoholic Beverages. Yeast is able to convert sugar into ethanol until the concentration reaches about 12-14% w/v, at which the yeast dies off. Consequently, it refers to the maximum alcohol content of wines, depending on the amount of sugar in the grapes. Its fermentation gets stopped before all the sugar has been fermented, the wine will be relatively sweet.

In some countries wines have been labelled 'dry' when they are having less than 8g carbohydrate per litre; less than 4g/l is labelled 'suitable for diabetics'; 25-40g/ medium; and sweet wines contain more than 45g/l.

Fortified wines are having extra alcohol added as 'spirit' of as brandy.

Alcoholism. An illness in which alcohol is drunk in large quantities resulting in dependence on it, damage to the liver and death.

Aldehydes. A large class of organic substances which are derived from primary alcohols by oxidation, and containing the grouping—CHO. For example, acetaldehyde, benzaldehyde.

Aldose. The general name for monosaccharides with an aldehyde (—CHO) as functional group.

Aldosterone. Hormone which is secreted by the adrenal cortex and controls the excretion of salt and water through the kidneys.

Ale. Beer.

Aleurone Layer. Refers to single layer of large cells under the bran coat and outside the endosperm of cereal grains; about 3% by weight of the grain, rich in protein. Botanically part of the endosperm but during milling remains attached to the inner layer or bran.

It is having about 20% of the thiamin, 30% of the riboflavin and 50% of the nicotinic acid of the grain.

Alewives. River herrings which, are mostly used for canning after salting.

Algae. Refers to the sub-group of the division of plants termed Thallophyta which show no differentiation into root, stem and leaf. They are mainly aquatic, and include seaweeds such as dulse and Irish moss, which have long been eaten by man.

Unicelluar varieties have been grown experimentally as novel sources of foods; these include Chlorella, Scenedesmus and Spirulina.

Protein, content 50-60% of dry weight.

Alginates. Refers to salts of alginic acid found as the free acid and calcium salt in many seaweeds. Alginic acid is a polysaccharide complex built from mannuronic acid units.

Salts like iron, magnesium and ammonium alginates from viscous solutions. The hold large amounts of water and are useful as thickeners, stabilisers, and gelling, binding and emulsifying agents in ice-cream, synthetic cream. The propyl glycol ester is used under the trade name of 'manucol ester'.

Alimentary Canal. The term used for the digestive tract, comprising, in man, mouth, oesophagus, stomach, duodenum, and small and large intestines.

Alimentary Pastes. Shaped dried Doughs which are made from semolina or wheat flour with water, and sometimes egg and milk. The dough is partly dried in hot air, then more slowly.

Macaroni-tubular-shaped, about 1/4 inch diameter; at 3/4 inch is called fovantini or maccaroncelli; at 1/2 inch, zitoni.

Spaghetti is solid rod about 3/32 inch diameter; vermicelli is a third of this thickness.

Noodles are shaped into sheets or ribbons.

Farfals are ground, granulated or shredded.

Alkaloids. Unspecific term originally used (Meissner, 1819) for basic nitrogen-containing compounds of plant origin. Infact some substances classed as alkaloids are not basic (e.g. colchicine) and are synthesised in animal tissues (phenylalkylamines and indoles). A pharmacological definition includes naturally occurring organic bases which are having marked pharmacological effects in animals (about 200 such compounds are known). Many are found in plant foods such as potato, tomato (Solanum alkaloids), ergot, animal foods (tetrodotoxin) in puffer fish, tetramine in shellfish, decarboxylated amino acids (tryptamine, tryamine, histamine); a number are used in drug treatment, such as morphine, colchicine, quinine, atropine.

Alkalosis. Refers to decrease in the acid-base ratio in the blood .plasma, or an increase in its buffering power. Causes may be excessive loss of carbon dioxide; excessive intake of base, as in antacid drugs; loss of gastric juice by vomiting; high intake of sodium or potassium salts of weak organic acids.

Alkannet. (alkanet, alkannim, aikanna) Colouring which is obtained from. root of Anchusa tintcoria (Alkana tincteria); legally permitted in food in most countries; colouring principle is alkannin. Insoluble in water but soluble in alcohol and ether. Blue in alkalies, blue with lead, crimson with tin, violet with iron. Used for colouring fats, cheese, essences (and interior port wine). Also known as orcanellà.

Allantoin. Oxidation product of uric acid. It is end-product of purine metabolism in most mammals except man and the anthropoid apes (where it is uric acid).

Allergen. A nontoxic substance or particle which causes slight or severe illness (food allergy in people sensitive to it. Many food compounds have been suggested to be allergens.

Allergy. Refers to an abnormal tissue reactivity after exposure to a foreign antigen which is caused by reaction with immunoglobulins in the tissues which results in the release of histamine, causing the clinical effects. Many people are sensitive (i.e. show a physiological reaction to various foods, but it is necessary to examine the immunological reaction before allergy can be distinguished from other forms of food intolerance. Milk, eggs, cheese and wheat are usually the causes of allergy, but almost all foods have been implicated.

Allicin. Sulphur compound which is responsible for the flavour of garlic.

Allinson Bread. A whole-wheat bread named after Allinson, who advocated its use in England at the end of the nineteenth century, as did Graham in the United States (thus, Graham bread).

Allolactose. Refers to a sugar, which may be a modification of lactose, which, together with gynolactose, has been claimed to be found in human milk.

Allotriophagy. Unnatural desire for foods; alternative words, cissa, cittosis and pica.

Alloxan. Refers to pyrimidine derivative that is able to induce diabetes when given orally or by injection, by damaging the islets of Langerhans (that part of the pancreas which secretes insulin).

Alloxan Diabets. Experimental diabets which get caused by alloxan.

Alloxanine. Three-ring structure, the central part of riboflavin. The latter is dimethyl-ribity-isoalloxazine.

Allspice. Refers to dried fruits of the evergreen Pimenta officinalis. It is also known as pimento or Jamaican pepper (differs from pimiento). The name 'allspice' derives from the volatile oil which has an aroma similar to a mixture of cloves, cinnamon and nutmeg. Used to flavour meat products.

Allysine. Semi-aldehyde of amino-adipic acid, formed in connective tissue by oxidative deamination of peptide-bound lysine.

Almond, Sweet. Ripe seeds of Prunus amygdalus var. dulcis: yields sweet almond oil.

Almond, Oil Bitter. Refers to essential oil from seeds of almond tree (Prunus amygdalus) or apricot tree (Prunus armeniaca). It is mostly manufactured from the apricot. 95% benzaldehyde, with hydrocyanic acid and bensaldehyde cyandydrin. When freed from hydrocyanic acid, is used as flavour, in perfumes and in cosmetics.

Aloe. Dried juice of leaves of Aloe perryi: It finds used in medicine. It is having a glycoside, aloe-emodin or rhabarberone, aloe oil, and aloin or barbaloin.

Alpha-laval Centrifuge. Refers to a continuous bowl centrifuge which is used for separating liquids of different densities for clarifying. Widely used for cream separation.

Aluminium. One of the most abundant elements in Nature. It is found in animal and plant tissues in traces but has not been shown to be essential to either.

'Alum' baking powders, in which sodium aluminium sulphate was the acid constituent, to be used.

'Silver' beads used to decorate confectionery may be coated with either silver foil or an aluminium copper alloy.

ALV. Available lysine value.

Alveographe. Refers to measures stretching quality of dough as index of protein quality for baking. A standard disc of dough is blown into a bubble and the pressure curve and bursting pressure measured; gives the stability, extensibility and strength.

Amama. Refers to trade name (Glaxo Laboratories) for a protein- rich baby food based on casein (1 part) and groundnut flour (10 parts) obsolete.

Amaranth. Burgundy-red colour which is fast to light. It is the trisodium salt of 1 (4-sulpho-lnaphthylazo 0-2-naphthol-3, 6-disulphonic acid).

Ambergris. Morbid concretion which is obtained from the intestine of the spern whale. Contains cholesterol, ambrein, benzoic acid. Appears as a mottled or striped grey-brown or black wax. Used in drugs and perfume.

Amberlite. Group of polystyrene resins which are used to absorb specific radicals from solutions. The sulphonic acid derivative, strongly acidic (IR 120), and the carboxylic acid, weakly acidic (IRC 150), are used for cation exchange; basic types used for anion exchange (IR4B, 1R45, IRA400). It is mainly used for water softening, mental recovery, purification of chemicals, chemical analysis, particularly amino acids.

Ames Test. Bacterial test system for mutagenic potential of substances (including food additives).

Amino Acid. It is characterised by an amino group and an acid group attached to the same carbon atom. Proteins are made of combinations of large numbers of amino acids of twenty different kinds. Eight of these amino acids must be provided in the diet—i.e., the essential amino acids e.g., lysine, methionine, valine, tryptophan, threonine, leucine, isoleucine and phenylalanine.. Possibly arginine and histidine are essential for infants. The remaining twelve can be synthesised in the body so long as a source of nitrogen is available in the diet. These include the non-essential amino acids: histidine, glycine, arfinine, alanine, aspartic acid, glutamic acid, proline, hydrodyproilne, serine cysteine and tyrosine.

Amino Acid Profile. Amino acid composition of a protein.

Amino Acids, Antiketogenic. Refer to those which get metabolised to glucose. They are glycine, alanine, serine, cystine, aspartic acid, glutamic acid, arginine, proline and hydropxyproline.

Amino Acids, Ketogenic. Refer to those which are metabolised to aceto-acetic acid (ketone bodies). They are leucine, isoleucine, phenylalanine and tyrosine.

Aminogram. Diagrammatic representation of the amino acid composition of a protein.

Aminopeptidase. Refers to an enzyme of the pancreatic juice which splits polypeptides to dipeptides. Removes the terminal unit of the Polypeptide chain at the end at which the amino radical is free; hence, is an exopeptidase.

Aminopterin. Aminopteroyglutamic acid which is specific antagonist to folic acid.

Ammonotelic. Descriptive of animals that are able to excrete their waste nitrogen as ammonia e.g., various worms, leeches, molluses, sea urchins, fish.

APM. See Adnosine Nucleotides.

Amydon. Starchy material which is made by steeping wheat flour in water and drying the starch sediment in the sun; used for many centuries for thickening broths.

Amygdalin. Glucoside in almonds, apricot and cherry stones. It is hydrolysed by the enzyme emulsin to glucose, hydrocyanic acid and benzaldehyde. The benzaldehyde provides the characteristic odour.

Amylases. Refer to enzymes that hydrolyse starch and glycogen to maltose.

Alpha-amylase, or dextrinogenic amylase, is able to

break starch down to small dextrin-like molecules and does not proceed to maltose.

Beta-amylase, or maltogenic amylase, is specific for the 1,4- alphaglucosidic linkages of starch any liberated maltose. Complete degradation of starch requires the attack of both these enzymes. Salivary amylase and pancreatic amylase in animals behave like the alpha-amylase. It is also known as diataste.

Amylodyspepsia. Inability to digest starch.

Amylograph. Measures the viscosity of flour paste as it is made to heat from 25 °C to 90°C (the same temperature rise as in baking) and serves as a measure of the diastatic activity of the flour.

Amyloins. Carbohydrates that are complexes of dextrins with varying proportions of maltose.

Amylolptic. General adjective applied to enzymes that are able to split starch into soluble products.

Amylopectin. Starch is having 20-25% amylose and the remainder amylopectin.

Amylose is having 1,4, alpha-inked glucose units and gives a pure blue with iodine. Amylopectin is a branched structure built up of 20-24 glucoside units linked 1,4, and gives a purplish colour with iodine.

Amylopsin. See Pancreatic amylase.

Amylose. The straight chain form of the starch polymer. It is quite soluble but forms crystals in some conditions, e.g., starch retrogradation.

Anablosis. Suspended animation (with stoppage of respiration and the heart-beat), which is caused by freezing or freezing and drying, as achieved, for example, by Alaskan and Siberian insects during cold spells.

Anabolism. The building of new molecules and macromolecules inside the cell using the energy and building block compounds produced by catabolism.

Anaemia. Means a shortage of red blood cells. It is caused by dietary shortage of Iron (nutritional iron-deficiency anaemia), by deficiency of the various vitamins involved in the formation of red blood cells, by lack of intrinsic factor (pernicious anaemia) leading to failure to absorb vitamin B_{12} (pernicious anaemia); primary cause is often chronic loss of blood due to intestinal damage caused by parasites.

Anaerobes. Refers to micro-organisms that grow in the absence of oxygen. Obligate anaerobes fail to survive in the presence of oxygen. Facultative anaerobes normally grow in oxygen but -can also grow in its absence.

Anaerobic. Of respiration which does not use, oxygen. Also of organisms whose respiration is anaerobic.

Analysis, Gastric. Fractional test meal.

Analysis, Proximate. The term used for an analysis for the major ingredients, usually nitrogen (as a measure of the protein), and fat and ash (as a measure of the mineral salts); these are added together and subtracted from 100 to give what is called 'carbohydrate by difference'. The latter may be corrected for crude fibre.

Anchovy. A fish, Engraulis encrasicholus. It is prepared semipreserved with 10-12% salt and sometimes benzoic acid.

Angostura. Essential oil which is distilled from the bark of Galipeacusparia. Contains galipol, cadinene, galipene and pinene; used in preparation of bitters and liqueurs.

Angstrom Unit. One ten-millionth part of a millimetre , or one ten-thousandth part of a micro; symbol A.

Angular stomatitis. Refers to an affection of the skin at the angles of the mouth, characterised by heaping up on epithelium into ridges, giving the appearance of fissures; a symptom of riboflavin deficiency but also a symptom of other diseases.

Anhydrovitamin A. Refers to a form of retinol in which the OH groups has been removed by treatment with HCL, with a corresponding shift in the double bonds. One incorrectly called cyclised or spurious vitamin A. Has very slight biological activity. When fed in large doses to rats, a more active material called rehydrovitamin A is obtained.

Animal Protein Factor. Name assigned to certain growth

factor or factors which were found to be present in animal but not vegetable proteins. Vitamin B_{12} was identified as one of these.

Aniseed (anise). Refers to the dried fruit of Pimpinella anisum (parsley family). Chief component of the volatile oil is anethole (methoxypropeny benzene). The seed finds use to flavour baked goods, meet products and drinks.

Anisette. Liqueur which is based on aniseed.

Annatto. Also called bixin or butter colour; colour from seed-pods of Bixa orellana. It is used for colouring butter and cheese (not margarine); legally permitted. Contains orellin, of minor importance. Soluble in water, and bixin, the major colour, insoluble in water. Also used to dye cotton and silk and in wood stains.

Anormers. A pair of stereosomers related to each other in the same way as alpha and beta glucose are related, are called anomers.

Anorectic Drugs. (Anorexigenic drugs) Refer to drugs that depress the appetite and are used an aid to weight reduction—e.g., amphetamine (or dextro-amphetamine or dexedrine), preludin (phenmetrazine hydrochloride), Tenuate (d ethylpropion).

Anorexia Nervosa. A phychological illness resulting in great loss of weight due to refusal to eat.

Anosmla. Lack or impairment of sensitivity to odour stimuli.

Aneserine. Beta-alanyl methylhistidine. It is a dipetide originally isolated from muscle. It is found in muscle of mammals, fishes and birds; function unknown.

Antabuse. Tetra-ethyl thiuramdisulphide. A drug which is used in the treatment of alcoholism. The drug alone has no effect, but if alcohol is subsequently taken, it gives rise to headache, palpitation, nausea and vomiting.

Antacids. Bases of buffers that are able to neutralise acid. These are used generally in relation to the partial neutralisation of Stomach acidity. Substances such as magnesium carbonate, sodium bicarbonate, magnesium hydroxide, glycine, etc., are used.

Anthocyanins. Voilet, red and blue water-soluble colouring matter of many fruits, flowers and leaves. Consist of glucose plus anthocyanidins (these consist of two 6-membered carbon rings containing one oxygen atom). Examples include delphinidin, pelarogonidin, cyanidin. Can attack iron and tin and cause trouble in canned foods.

Anthocyanidins. A group of related chemicals which contain a number of aromatic rings and hydroxyl (-OH) functional groups Anthocyanidins combine with sugars through the formation of glycosidic bonds to produce the coloured anthocyanins.

Anthoxanthins. Alternative name for flavonoids.

Antibiotics. Substances which are produced by living organisms. These inhibit the growth of other organisms. Classic example is penicilin, produced by the mould Pecillium notatum, which inhibits bacteria and is used to control infections by susceptible bacteria.

When they are added to the diet of animals in small quantities (a few grams per tonne of food), many antibiotics stimulate growth, possibly by increasing the efficiency of food absorption or by controlling mild infections. To prevent the development of antibiotic-resistant strains of bacteria, the use as feed additives is limited to varieties not used therapeutically such as risin. The latter also finds use as a food preservative.

Antibodies. The proteins which are formed in the blood in response to 'foreign' proteins-antigens. These proteins are immuno-globulins of which there are five types, 1gM, G, A, D and E.

Immunity to infection is due to the presence in the blood of antitoxins (specific antibodies) formed in response to the initial infection with bacterial antigens.

Anti-eaking Agents. Added to powder foodstuffs to prevent caking e.g., small amounts of anhydrous disodium hydrogen phosphate added to salt or sugar: aluminium carbonate in table salt; calcium silicate in baking powder.

Anticoagulants. With reference to blood, substances that do not allow clotting by interfering with the mechanism. Oxalate and citrate are anticoagulants, as they combine with the calcium which is needed; discoumarin and heparn inhibit the formation of prothrombin, needed to release fibrin from fibrinogen; hirudin inactivates the thrombin.

Antidiuretics. Drugs that are able to reduce the rate of formation of urine, i.e., reduce water loss from the body.

Antienzymes. Refer to substances that specifically inhibit the action of digestive enzymes produced by the lining of the digestive tract, secreted by intestinal parasites, found in raw legumes (antitypsin, antiamylase); destroyed by heat.

Antifoaming Agents. Octanol (capry alchol), sulphonated oils, silicones. They reduce foaming often caused by the presence of dissolved protein or other stabiliser.

Antigalactics. Substances that are able to suppress the secretion of milk.

Anti-grey Hair Factor. Absence of either para-aminobenzoic acid or pantothenic acid can bring about the loss of hair colour in rats; not related to loss of hair pigment in human beings.

Anti-mould Agents. See Antimycotics.

Antimycotics. Refers to substances that are able to inhibit mould growth, such as sodium and calcium propionate, methyl hydroxybenzoate, quaternary ammonium chloride, sodium benzoate, sorbic acids

Antioxidants. Substances that are able to retard the oxidative rancidity of fats—e.g., propyl gallate, octyl gallate, dodecyl gallate, butykated hydroxyanisole (BHA) and butylated hydroxytoluene (BHT). Many fats, particularly vegetable lils, contain naturally occurring antioxidants, such as tocopherol, which protect the oils from rancidity for a limited period.

Antisialagongues. Substances that are able to arrest the flow of saliva.

Anti-soattering Agents. Added to fats used in frying—e.g., lecithin, sucrose esters (laurates and stearates), and sodium sulphoacetate derivates of mono-and diglycerides. They function by preventing the coalescence of water droplets.

Anti-Staling Agents. Refers to the substances that retard the staling of baked products, and also soften the crumb—e.g., sucrose stearate, polyoxyethylene monostearate, glyceryl monosterate, stearoyl tartrate.

Antivitamins. Refers to substances that interfere with the function of vitamins or destroy them. Dicoumarol in spoiled sweet clover inhibits function of vitamin K; thiaminse in raw fish destroys thiamin; the drug methotrezate inhibits folate.

AOM. Active oxygen method.

Apastia. Refusal to take food as an expression of mental disorder.

Aphagosis. Inability to eat.

Apoferritin. Refers to the protein part of ferritin, the iron storage complex in the intestinal mucosal cells.

Appollinaris Water. An alkaline, highly aerated water which is containing sodium chloride and calcium, sodium and magnesium carbonates.

Aporinosis. Term for any disease which arises due to deficiency of an element in diet. (Greek aporos, scarce.)

Apporrhegama. Ptomaine or other toxic substance split off from an amino acid during the bacterial decomposition of a protein.

Aposia. Absence of feeling of thirst.

Apositia. Aversion for food.

Appertisation. Term applied by the French to the process of destroying all the micro-organisms of significance in food, i.e, commercial sterility; a few organisms remain alive but are quiescent. (Named after Nicholas Appert.)

Appel. Fruit of many species of Malus sylvestris (origin of name of malic acid).

Analysis per 100g : 84g water, 2g dietary fibre (3.7 in 100g skin), 46 kcal (0.2 MJ); only 3mg vitamin C in eating apples, 15-20 mg in cooking apples.

Appa Butter. Refers to apple that has been boiled in an

open kettle to a thick consistency. Similar to apple sauce but darker in colour, because of the prolonged boiling.

Appel, Jack. American name for apple brandy; distilled cider, also known as Calvados.

Apple Liquid. Refers to American preparation of apple juice plus pulverised apple pulp in suspension.

Apple Nuggets. Refers to crisp granules of apple of low moisture content. Dehydrated apples of 24% moisture content are cut into small cubes and dried down 2% moisture; used to make apple sauce.

Apricot. Fruit of Prunus armeniaca.

Analysis per 100g (without stones): 87g water, 7g sugar, 2g dietary fibre, 1000-25000g carotene, 7mg vitamin C, 30 kcal (0.IMJ). Dried apricots, per 100g: 15g water, 43g sugar, 24 dietary fibre, 4 mg iron, 3000-40000 μg carotene, trace of vitamin C.

Arachidonic Acid. Refers to a straight-chain fatty acid which is containing twenty carbon atoms and four double bonds (a tetraene). Found only in animal fats, e.g,. brain, liver, egg yolk.

Arachin. One of the globulin proteins from the peanut. It gets precipitated by 40% saturated ammonium sulphate from a salt extract of peanut. Conarachin can be precipitated from the residue by 85% saturated ammonium sulphate.

Arachis Oil. Peanut or groundnut oil which is extracted from Arachis hypogea-earthnut, groundnut, monkey nut, peanut. About 50% oleic acid. 30% linoleic acid, less than 1% linolenic acid.

Arginase. Enzyme that is able to hydrolyse arginine to urea and ornithine, the last stage of urea synthesis from the aminogroups of the amino acids. Present in most animal cells.

Arginine. Chemically, aminoguanido valeric acid. Dibasic aminoacid that is non-essential to adult man. Since it is partly essential to growing rats (growth only 80% of optimum in its absence), it may similarly be partly essential to children. It is essential to the chick.

Argol. The term used for the crust of crude cream of (tartar potassium acid tartrate) which forms on the sides of wine vats (also called wine stone). White argol from white grapes, red argol from red. 50-85% potassium hydrogen tartrate and 6-12% calcium tartrate used in vinegar fermentation, as mordant in dyeing, and in the manufacture of tartaric acid.

Ariboflavinosis. Deficiency of riboflavin (vitamin B_2) which is chatacterised by swollen, cracked, bright red lips (Cheilosis), enlarged, tender, magenta-red tongue (glossitis), cracking at the corners of the mouth (angular stomatitis) and congestion of the blood vessels of the conjunctiva.

Armenian Bole (ferric oxide). Occurs naturally as hematite or obtained by heating ferrous sulphate, etc. It finds use in metallurgy, polishing compounds, paint pigment and as a food colour.

Arrowroot. Tuber of the West Indian plant Maranta arundinacea. It is mainly used to prepare arrowroot starch, the most refined of all feculas. The starch is having only a trace of protein (0.2%) and is free from vitamins. It finds use in bland, lowsalt and protein-restricted diets and, unfortunately, as an infant food in some West Indian islands.

Arsanilic Acid. Used to stimulate growth in poultry.

Arsenic. Toxic chemical believed to react with cellular sulphydryl groups. It can accumulate in fish and shellfish and in crops treated with arsenical pesticides.

Ascorbic Acid. Vitamin C. It is also called L-xyloascorbic acid, in distinction from D-araboscorbic acid (isoacorbic acid or erythorbic acid), which is having only slight vitamin C activity.

Erythorbic acid has strong reducing properties, and is used as an antioxidant in foods and to preserve the red colour of fresh or preserved meats.

Physiological properties of ascorbic acid are described under vitamin C.

Ascorbic Acid Browning. The process by which ascorbic

acid breaks down to give brown-coloured products. This reaction can happen under both aerobic and anaerobic conditions.

Ascorbic, Acid Oxides. Refers to plant enzyme that oxidises ascorbic acid to the dehydro form. In the living tissue it appears to get separated from the vitamin, but in the wilting leaf or, for example, in shredded cabbage, the enzyme comes into contact with its substrate and there is a rapid destruction of the vitamin.

Ascorbin Stearate. Ester of ascorbic acid (vitamin C) and stearic acid. It is fat-soluble form of the vitamin which finds use as an antioxidant at concentrations around 0.1%.

Ascorbonyl Palmitate. Ester of ascorbic acid and palmitic acid which is an anti-staling agent in bakery products. Amounts of 0.1-0.4% by weight of the flour retard staling for 2-4 days.

Aseptic. Means without contamination by micro-organisms.

Aseptic Filling. Refers to filling containers (cans) with food that has already been sterilised and so must be maintained under aseptic conditions. Continuous sterilisation as the food passes along narrow pipes permits more rapid heating, with less effect on the quality of the food.

Ash. The part of a food which remains after all the organic substances have been burnt. Ash is used as a measure of the amount of inorganic compounds in the food.

Asparagine. Refers to an amide of the amino acid aspartic acid; serves in plants as a store of ammonia. During the growth of seedlings ketonic acids are formed during photosynthesis, and these are aminated to amino acids at the expense of the ammonia in asparagine.

Asparagus. Refers to young shoot of Asparagus officinalis. Analysis per 100g; protein 1.4g, fat 0.1g. Ca 14mg, Fe 0.6mg, kcal 14 (60kJ), vitamin A 220µg. vitamin B_1 0.11mg, vitamin B_2 0.13mg, nicotine acid 0.9mg, vitamin C 22mg.

Aspartamate. Artificial sweetener, N-L-asparty-L-phenylalanine methyl ester. It is 200 times as sweet as 4% solution of sucrose. It is stable for only a limited time in solution (some months) when it breaks down to diketopreperazine derivatives. It is used in soft drinks, dessert mixes, as 'table-top sweetener' etc.

Aspartic Acid. Refers to non-essential amino acid; succinic acid (dibasic). Its amide is asparagine.

Aspartyl-phenylalanine Methyl Ester. Dipeptide ester.

Aspergillus. Moulds; takadiastase.

Aspic Jelly. A clear jelly which is made from fish, chicken or meat stock, sometimes with added gelatin, flavoured with lemon, taragon vinegar, sherry, peppercorns and vegetables, and used to glaze meat or game, among other foods. Name derived from the herb espic or spikenard.

Assimilation. The process by which digested food is absorbed through the wall of the small intestine into the blood steam.

Astaxanthin. A carotenoid pigment which is responsible for the pink colour of salmon muscle.

Astringency. Literally, a 'drawing together'; property of foods, especially unripe fruits and cider apples, thought to be due to the destruction of the lubricant properties of the salvia and contraction of epithelial tissues of the tongue by precipitation by tannins, which see.

Atmungsferment. Name given by Warburg to the respiratory enzyme, later called cytochrome oxidase.

ATP. Adenosine Triphosphate. The main store of chemical energy in the cell. It contains three phosphate groups each of which is bonded to the next by a high energy bond. ATP is the product of respiration.

Atwater Factors. Factors used to calculate the energy available from foodstuffs after allowing for the losses of digestion and the incomplete combustion of the nitrogen part of proteins. The complete heat of combustion of proteins is 5.7, of fats 9.4 and of carbohydrates 4.1 kcal/g; Atwater factors are, respectively, 4,9 and 4 kcal/g.

Aubergine. Also known as egg plant Solanum melongena. It is native of S.E. Asia. It is 3-5 inches in diameter and up to 12 inches long, purple in colour. Its composition per 100g is carbohydrate 6g, protein 1.4g, vitamin B_1 0.06mg, B_2 0.05mg nicotinic acid 0.8mg, vitamin C 5mg.

Aurantiamarin. Glucoside which is present in the albedo of the bitter orange. It is partly responsible for the flavour.

Aureomycin. See Tetracyclines.

Autoclave. Refers to a vessel in which high temperatures can be reached by using high pressure. An example of this is the domestic pressure cooker.

Autoclaves have two major purposes. The domestic pressure cooker permits cooking in a shorter time. The second major use is in sterilisation. Bacteria get destroyed more readily at these elevated temperatures, and autoclaves are used to sterilise food, for example in cans, and for sterilising instruments and dressings in surgery.

Autolysis. Process of self-digestion which is effected by the enzymes naturally present in the tissue. For example, tenderising of game while hanging is autolytic breakdown of connective tissue.

Auto-oxidation. The process by which triglycerides are oxidized. It is called auto-oxidation because once started, the process catalyses itself. It has three stages:

1. Invitation
2. Propagation and
3. Termination.

Autotrophes. Organisms that can synthesis their own tissues from simple inorganic salts, as distinct from heterotophes, which must be supplied with complex ready-made foods. Thus, plants are autotrophes, animals are heterotrophes. Bacteria can be of either type. Autotrophes are not involved in food spoilage: heterotrophic bacteria include pathogens and food-spoilage organisms.

Auxins. Refers to plant hormones which get produced in the growing buds, embryos and young leaves of plants, as well as many fungi and bacteria. They are organic acids—*e.g.,* indolyl acetic acid, indolyl butyic acid and naphthalene acetic acid. Used to stimulate root formation and control growth.

Available Carbon Dioxide. Banking power; flour, self-raising. The protein-bound lysine in which the end-amino group is free, so that after enzymic hydrolysis-digestion—the lysine is available for absorption. In contrast, when the end-amino group of the lysine is bound to a reducing sugar (Maillard reation) or by another linkage that cannot be hydrolysed during degestion, the lysine is unavailable. Such linkage get hydrolysed by acid digestion in vitro, so giving rise to a discrepancy between chemical and biological determination of protein quality.

Available Nutrients. In some foodstuffs nutrients shown to be present by chemical tests may not be available, or be only partly available, to the animal. For example, the calcium combined in phytin, and the lysine that is combined with sugar in the Maillard complex, are not available, as they cannot be liberated by the digestive enzymes.

Avenalin. Refers to the globulin protein present in oats.

Avenin. Refers to the glutelin protein present in oats.

Avicel. Trade name (American Viscose Co.) for microcrystalline alpha-cellulose-natural cellulose partly hydrolysed with acid and reduced to a fine power. Disperses in water and has the properties of a gum; used to make oily foods such as cheese, peanut butter, as well as syrups and honey, into dry granular powders; also used in sauces and dressings.

Avidin. Refers to protein in white of egg which combines with vitamin H (biotin) and renders it unavailable to the body. It gets inactivated in cooked eggs.

Avitaminosis. Absence of a vitamin; may be used specifically, as avitaminosis A.

Avocado (alligator pear). Refers to fruit of Persea americana. Unusual among fruits in its high fat content, 17-27%.

Analysis per 100g: 69g water 4g protein 22g fat, 1,8g carbohydrate, 5-30 mg vitamin C, 220 kcal (920 kJ). 7-14% of the fat is linoletic acid.

Axerol, Axerophthol. Suggested names for vitamin A but is not used.

Azaserine. Diazoacetyl derivative of the non-essential amino acid serine. Interferes with the metabolism of serine and acts as an anti-cancer agent.

Azlon. Name given to textile fibres which are produced from proteins, such as casein, zein.

Azo Dyes. Refers to a group of compounds which are formed by combining a diazonium salt to an aromatic amino or hydroxy-compound; they contain two nitrogen atoms combined together and are all strongly coloured. Some are permitted in foods.

Azotobacter. Genus of bacteria of family Bacteriaceae, they can use atmospheric nitrogen and synthesise nitrogenous tissue from it.

B

Babassu Oil. Edible oil which is isolated from the Braxillian palm nut; similar to coconut oil, and used in food, soap and cosmetics.

Babcock Test. Refers to a test for fat in milk. The sample is mixed with sulphuric acid in a Babcock bottle, centrifuged, diluted and recentrifuged. The level of the fat in the neck of the bottle is read off.

Bacalao. South American name for klipfish.

Bacitracin. In a antibiotic which is isolated from an organism of the Bacillus subtilis group; w polypeptide.

Bacon. Refers to the smoked and cured meat made from pig-back, sides and bellt (old French of pig).

The pig meat is produced by curing the carcass or portions of meat in salt solutions (p.22) called brine (p.163). The brine normally contains 25-30% by weight of sodium chloride, 2.54% potassium nitrate and often salt-tolerant backeteria which convent potassium nitrite. The nitrite is broken down to nitric oxide which combines with myoglobin to give the pink colour of bacon. Curing can take several days.

Gammon (usually top of hind leg), analysis per 100g: 25g protein, 19g fat. 270 kcal (1.1 MJ).

Rasher (single slice) can be having up to 40% fat. Pig meat is exceptionally rich in thiamin, containing about 0.5 rug per 100g (upto 1mg in lean meat), about ten ties as much as bed; riboflavin (0.2-0.3) and niacin (3-g mg) are similar in amounts to those of other meats.

Bacteria. A large group of micro-organisms which can be both harmful and helpful to man. They are single-called but contain no nucleus. Many are pathogenic and cause food poisoning as well as food spoilage but some live in the intestines of man and provide benefits such as producing vitamins *e.g.* biotin and others are useful in termenting *e.g.* yoghurt. Bacteria are divided into four main classes; (1) coccus, (2) bacilus (3) vibrio, (4) spirillum.

Some bacteria, the so-called pathogens, produce toxins which bring about disease. Some are spore-formers and in this form they are more resistant to heat and sterilising agents. Bacteria contain 45-85% dry matter as protein and are grown on petroleum residues, mathane or methanol for animal feed.

Bacterial Count. Plate count.

Bacteriophage. Refers to a group or viruses that attack bacteria. They are composed of nucleoprotein and capable of multiplying in host cells. They are smaller than bacteria and can pass through ordinary bacterial filters. Cause of considerable trouble in culture suspensions—*e.g.* in milk starter cultures, as these readily become infected with phages.

Bacterium Aceti. Acetobacter.

Bactofugation. Belgian process for removing bacteria from milk by high-speed centrifuging.

Bagasse. Mill residues from sugar-cane having the crushed stalks from which the juice has been expressed; 50% cellulose, 25% hemicelluloses, 25% lignin. Sometimes also applied to residues from other plants , such as beet. Used as fuel and as cattle feed, in preparation of paper and fibre board, and in manufacture of furfural.

Bain Marie. Double saucepan (French for water-bath).

Baking Additives. Materials which are added to flour products for a variety of purposes, including bleaching of the flour, aging (which see), seowing rate of staling, improving texture.

Baking Powder. A mixture that liberates carbon dioxide

when moistened or heated. Sodium bicarbonate is the source of CO_2 and an acidic substance is required, such as tartaric acid or acid salt, calcium acid phosphate, sodium pyrophosphate or sodium aluminum sulphate. Quick-acting powders are having tartrate and liberate CO_2 in the dough before heating; slow-acting powders contain phosphate and liberate most of the CO_2 during heating.

Must contain not less than 8% available, and not more than 1.5% residual, CO_2. Golden raising powder (similar but coloured yellow; formerly called egg-substitute) must contain not less than 6% available, and not more than 1.5% residual, CO_2.

Bal-ahar. A protein-rich baby food (22-26% protein) which is made in India from wheat flour, oil-seed flour and vegetables, with added vitamins and calcium.

Balance. With reference to diet, means net gain (positive balance) or loss (negative balance); used in reference to nitrogen, mineral salts, etc. When intake equals excretion, the body is in equilibrium with respect to the nutrient in question. Balanced diet is one containing all nutrients.

Balanced Diet. A diet in which each nutrient is supplied in the correct quantities relative to all other nutrients.

Balling. Refers to table of specific gravity published by von Balling in 1843, giving the weight of cane sugar in 100g of solution corresponding with s.g. determined at 17.5°C. It finds use in calculating the percentage extract in beer worts. It was corrected for slight inaccuracies by Plato, 1900. Extracts are referred to as percent Plato.

For s.g. greater than unity s.g.=200 divided by (200 minus scale reading): for s.g. less than unity s.g.=200 divided by (200 plus scale reading).

Ball Mill. Refers to a vessel in which material is ground by rolling heavy balls; used for hard materials.

Balmain Bug. A variety of lobster which is found in Australia.

Bambarra Groundnut. Voandzeia subterranea.

Resembles true groundnut but seeds are low in oil content. Seeds are hard and need soaking or pounting before cooking.

Analysis per 100g: 18g protein, 6g fat, 60g carbohydrate, 367 kcal (1.5MJ), 65mg Ca, 6mg Fe, 0.3 mg vitamin B_1, 0.1mg vitamin B_2, 2mg nicotinic acid.

Bamboo Shoots. Refers to thick, pointed shoots of Bambusa Vulgaris and Phyllostachys pubescens eaten in eastern Asia.

Analysis per 100g : 2.3g protein, 0.2g fat, 6g carbohydrate, 367kcal (0. 15MJ), 0.15mg vitamin B_1, 0-07mg vitamin B_2. 0.6mg nicotinic acid, 4mg vitamin C.

Banana. Fruit of genus Musa; but since the cultivated kinds have been sterile hybrid forms, they cannot be given exact species names. Dessert bananas are having a high sugar content (17-19%) and are eaten raw.

Analysis per 100g; 1 g protein, 0.3g fat, 27g carbohydrate, 116 kcal 0.49MJ), 0.5mg Fe, 30mg vitamin A, 0.05mg vitamin B_1, 0.05mg vitamin B_2, 0.7mg nicotinic acid, 10mg vitamin C. Sodium content is low, 1.2mg per 100g. so used in low-sodium diets.

Bana, False. Ensete Ventricosum. It is closely related to the banana; fruits are small and contain seeds (bananas are sterile and have no seeds); the rhizome and inner tissues of the stem are eaten after cooking (major food in S. Ethiopia).

Analysis of rhizome per 100g; 1.5g protein, 45g carbohydrate, 190 kcal (0.8MJ), 5mg Fe, 0.02mg vitamin B_1, 0.05mg. vitamin B_2, 0.2mg nicotinic acid, 0.5mg vitamin C.

Banana Figs. Bananas are split longitudinally and sun-dried without treating with sulphur dioxide. The product is dark in colour and sticky.

Bannock. Refers to flat round cake which is made of oat, rye or barely meal. It is baked on a hearth or griddle.

Pitcaithly bannock is type of almond shortbread containing caraway seeds and chopped peel.

Bap. Refers to a soft, white, flat, floury-coated Scottish breakfast roll.

Barbados Cherry. Cherry, West Indian.

Barbados Sugar. Sugar.

Bar Coding. A system by which packaged food products can be labelled with a code made up of vertical bars. The bars can represent various important facts about the product, e.g., its description and price. Bar codes are read by moving them over an automatic scanner connected to a computer. This allows control of the sale and stock of food products and eliminates human error.

Barding. See Larding.

Barfoed's Test. For all monosaccharides. Barfoed's solution is copper acetate in acetic acid, which gives a red precipitate of cuprous oxide with monosaccharides.

Barium meal. Refers to a meal having barium sulphate, which is opaque to X-rays, and allows examination of the shape and movements of the stomach for diagnostic purposes.

Barley. Refers to grain of Hordeum vulgare, of considerable importance as human and animal food and in brewing. It is one of the hardiest of cereals.

The whole grain with only the outer husk removed is termed as pot, scotch or hulled barley (this requires several hours cooking).

Pearl barley-most of the bran and germ removed, ash reduced from 2.5 to 1%, vitamin B_1 to one-tenth.

Analysis per 100g, protein 9g, fat 1.4g, Ca 20mg, Fe 0.7mg, vitamin $B_1$0.l5mg, vitamin B_2 0.08mg, nicotine acid 2.5mg.

Barley meal is ground hulled barley; barely flour is ground pearl barley; barley flakes are the flattened grain.

Barley, Malted. see Malt.

Barm. Refers to another name for yeast or leaven, or the froth on fermenting malt liquor.

Spon or virgin barm (short for apontaneous) is obtained by allowing 'wild yeast to fail into a sugar medium and multiply there.

Basal Metabolic Rate (BMR). If the body is at complete

rest, free from draughts, at moderate room temperature and 12-14 hours after a meal, energy is being used at the basal rate—the basal metabolism. This energy is required to maintain the heart beat, respiration, etc., but largely to maintain body temperature and the tension of the musics. BMR is therefore related to muscle mass and the surface area of the body. It is calculated from surface area of the body. It is calculated from surface area; the output per square meter varies with age and sex.

For male infants BMR has been 50-70 kcal per square meter per hour, falling steadily with age to 30-40 kcal at the age of 70, about 10% less for women.

Average BMR, about 1500 kcal (6MJ) per day. It has been under control of the thyroid gland, increased in fever and hyperthyroidism, and by administration of throxine or dried thyroid, and reduced when the throid is underactive.

Basic 7 Foods Plan. Division of foods into seven groups with the recommendation that some food from each group should be eaten every day, so ensuring a well-mixed diet.

Group 1, green and yellow vegetables. Group 2, oranges, tomato, grapefruit and raw salads. Group 3, potatoes and other vegetables and fruits. Group 4, milk and cheese. Group 5, meat, poultry, fish and eggs. Group 6, bread, flour, cereals. Group 7, butter, margrine.

Basil. May be one of four different types of herb, but the main one is the European sweet basil, Octimum basilicum. It finds use in seasoning.

Batata. Potato, sweet.

Bath Chap. Cheek and jawbones of the pig, which are salted and smoked.

Baume. A table of specific gravity which is used for salt solutions. For s.g. greater than unity, s.g. 145 divided by (145 minus degree Baume): for s.g. less than unity, s.g.= 140 divided by (130 plus degrees Baume).

Bdelygmia. Extreme lating for food.

Be. Abbreviation for degree Baume.

Beans. Refer to the seeds of a wide variety of leguminous plants.

Beans, Baked. Usually mature haricot beans, Phaseolus vulgaris, cooked by autoclaving.

Beans, Broad. Vicia faba.

Analysis after cooking, whole beans without pod, per 100g; water 84g. protein 4g, carbohydrate 7g, kcal 43 (176 kJ), Fe 1mg, nicotinic acid 3mg, vitamin C 15mg. Also known as horse bean.

Beans, Butter. Phaseolus lunatus.

Analysis after cooking, per 100g: water 70.5g, fat trace, protein 7g, carbohydrate 17g, kcal 93 (390 kJ), Fe 1.7mg. Also known as Lima bean (USA), curry bean, madagascar bean and sugar bean.

Beans, French. Phaseolus vulgaris, eaten unripe in the pod. Analysis after cooked pod and beans per 100g: water 95.5g, fat trace, protein 0.8g, carbohydrate 1.1g, kcal 7 (30 KJ), Fe 0.6mg carotine 600 µg, vitamin C 5mg. Mature bean has been the haricot bean.

Beans, Haricot. Ripe seeds of Phaseolus vulgaris (unripe seed is the French bean).

- Analysis of cooked bean per 100g : water 70g, fat trace, protein 6.6g, carbohydrate 16.6g, kcal 89 (370 kJ), Ca 65mg Fe 2.5mg. Also termed as Navy, pinto or snap beans (USA).

Beans Runner. Phaseolus multiflorus, eaten unripe with pod. Analysis after cooking, per 100g: water 93.6%, protein 0.8%, carbohydrate 0.9g, kcal 7 (30 kJ), Fe 0.6mg, carotene 300µg, nicotinic acid 0.5mg, vitamin C 5mg.

Beche-dr-mer. Sea slug, Stichopus japonicus, also called trepang; an occasional food in most parts of the world. Analysis per 100g: protein 22g, carbohydrate 1g, fat trace, Ca 120mg, Fe 1.4, kcal 94 (394 kJ).

Beetchwood Sugar. Xylose.

Beef. Flesh of ox; its composition varies with amount of fat present and the particular cut-*e.g.* brisket, rump, silverside, etc.

Dressed carcass, analysis per 100g raw; 280 kcal (1. I7MJ), 16g protein, 24g fat, 59g water, 1.9mg Fe, 3.3mg Zn, 0.05mg thiamin, 0.2mg riboflavin, 0.2mg vitamin E, 0.2mg vitamin B_6, 1 µg vitamin B_{12}. 4µg free folate, 0.5mg pantothenate; other vitamins present only in trace amounts.

Rump teak, fried, analysis per 100g; 250 kcal (1.0MJ) 29g protein, 15g fat, 56g water, 0.08mg thiamin, 0.35mg roboflavin, 5.5mg niacin, 0.33mg vitamin E, 0.3mg vitamin B_6 2µg vitamin B_{12}, 4µgfree folate, 0.8mg pantothenate; traces of other vitamins.

Beefalo. Refers to cross between bull and buffalo which can get fattened on range grass rather than requiring cereal and protein supplement.

Beef Tea. Refers to an extract of stewing beef prepared by simmering for 2-3 hours. Used to be for invalids, as the meat extractive stimulate the appetite.

Beer. An alcoholic beverage which is produced by fermentation of cereals. The first step in manufacture is malting of the barely. It is allowed to sprout, when the enzyme amylase develops and hydrolyses the starch to dextrins and maltos. The sprouted barley is dried and extracted with hot water (the process is called mashing) to produce wort. After the addition of hops for flavour the wort is allowed to ferment.

Ale is a light-coloured beer which is obtained by top fermentation and containing more alcohol and hops.

Porter is obtained from partly charred malt and is darker in colour is also a top fermentation.

Stout is similar to porter, but contains more extract and a higher alcohol content.

Lager is obtained by bottom fermentation, is low in alcohol content, is rich in extract and is aged after fermentation.

Most beers, ale and stout have 3.7% alcohol and 30-60kcal per 100ml.

Beestings. The term used for the first milk given by the cow after calving.

Beet Common Red. Root of Beta vulgaris.
Analysis per 100g, boiled; water protein 1.8g, fat trace, carbohydrate 100g, kcal 44 (185 kJ), Fe 0.7mg, Ca 30mg. carotene trace, vitamin B_1 0.02mg, vitamin B_2 0.04mg, nicotinic acid 0.06mg, vitamin C 5mg.

Beat Sugar. Refers to sucrose which is extracted from the sugar beet. It is identical with sucrose extracted from the sugar beet. It is identical with sucrose extracted from any other source.

Beeturia. The term used for the production of red-pigmented urine after eating beetroot; occurs in only one person in eight and not consistently. The colour is due to the pigment Betamin.

Beet Wine. A wine which gets produced by the usual alcoholic fermentation of sugar, but using yeast in the form of a clump of yeast and lactic bacteria. The clump rises and falls with bubbles or carbon dioxide produced; hence the 'bee'.

Bemax. Trade name (Vitamins Ltd) of a wheat germ preparation.
Analysis per 100g; protein 27.8g, fat 9.3g, carbohydrate 44.7g, Ca 54mg, Fe 7.7mg, kcal 368 (1.55MJ), vitamin B_1 1.6mg, vitamin B_2 0.7mg, nicotinic acid 7mg.

Benedictine. French liquer which was invented and manufactured by Benedictine monks at the Abbey of Fecamp; approximately 30% alcohol, 30% sugar, 300kcal (1.3 MJ) per 100ml.

Benedict-roth Spirometer. The equipment used to measure the amount of carbon dioxide (CO_2) from which the amount of energy used can be determined.

Benedict's Test. A test used for reducing sugars; solution of copper-sulphate, sodium citrate and sodium carbonate which gives a green, yellow or red precipitate on heating with a reducing agent, depending on the amount present. Benedict's quantitative reagent also includes potassium thiocyanate and potassium ferrocyanide.

Benniseed. See Sesame.

Benzidine Test. Very sensitive test for blood. The substance under test is added to saturated solution of benzidine in glacial acetic acid, followed by hydrogen peroxide. A blue or green colour is positive.

Benzoate. Benezoic acid.

Benzoic Acid. C_6H_5COOH. Free acid and salts are used as food preservative, especially in foods such as pickle and sauces; occurs naturally in cranberry and bilberry and in high concentrations in cloudberry. Excreted in urine conjugated with glycine as hippuric acid.

Bergamot. An orange, Citrus bergamia, which is confined almost entirely to the province of Calabria in S. Italy. Used only for extraction of the peel oil for perfumery.

Beriberi. Result of a severe vitamin B_1 deficiency. It is common in the Far East, where white (polished) rice forms the bulk of the died and vitamin B_1 is poorly supplied.

There have been two forms of beriberi: the wet form, where oedema is present, and dry beriberi, where there is extreme emaciation. In both forms there is a degeneration of the nerves affecting the lower limbs first, gastrointestinal disorders, mental symptoms, an enlarged heart with an increased rate of beat; death ultimately is caused from cardiac failure.

Berries. Botanical name for fruits in which seeds get embedded in pulpy tissue-*e.g.*, strawberry, currant, tomato.

Betaine. Trimethylglycine. Found in beetroot and cottonseed; also known as lycine and oxyneurine (obsolete names). Related to choline; possesses labile methyl groups.

Beta-oxidation. Refers to one of the routes of fatty acid metabolism. Oxidation at the carbon atom beta to the carboxyl group of the fatty acid *(i.e.* next but one), with the formation of the betakeotonic acid. Acetic acid then splits off, leaving a fatty acid two carbon atoms shorter than the original.

Betel. Leaf of the creeper Piper betel or betel. It is chewed in some parts of the world for its stimulating effect (due to presence of the alkaloids recoline and guvacoline). The leaves are chewed with nuts of the areca palm, Areca catechu. Which is therefore often termed as the betel palm, and the nut is termed as the betel nut.

Bazoar. Refers to a hard ball of undigested food which forms in the ach and can cause intestinal obstruction. Foods with a high content of indigestible pectin such as orange pith can form bezoars if swallowed without chewing.

BHA. Butylated hydroxyanisole.

BUT. Butylated hydroxytoluene.

Bifidus Factor. Name given to a substance in human milk, apparently a glucosamine, which stimulates the growth of Lactobacillus bifidus in the infant's intestine, which increases the formation of lactic and acetic acids and lowers the pH of the stools. Synthetic equivalent is lactulose, which see.

Biffins. Apples that have been peeled, partly backed then pressed end dried.

Bigaradier. French term for the bitter orange.

Bilberry. Berry of shrub of species Vacinium. Variously named whortleberry, blaeberry (Iceland), windberry, huckleberry. Not cultivated but grows wild.

Analysis per 100g: water 76.6-87, protein 0.7g, free acid 1.1- 1.7g. sugar 3.8-6.8g, pentosans, etc., 0.6-1 Ag, fibre 3.7-12.0g, ash 0.3-1.0g.

Bile. A liquid which is produced by the liver and stored in the gall bladder which is embedded in the liver. It consists of bile salts (sodium glycocholate and sodium taurocholate), bile pigments (bilirubin and biliverdin) and cholesterol. The bile slats play a part in the digestion of fats, as they decrease the surface tension and aid the formation of a fine emulsion of fat. The bile pigments are waste products which are formed from the breakdown of haemoglobin and they are excreted in the faeces.

The bile travels from the gall bladder to the duodenum via the bile duct.

Bile Salts. Bile.

Bilirubin. Refers to one of the bile pigments which is formed by the degradation of haemoglobin; a reduction product of biliverdin.

Biliverdin. One of the bile pigments which is formed by the degradation of haemoglobin; a reduction.

Biltong. Dried meat strips (South Africa). The meat has been cut in 2 inch strips, 2-3 feet long, along the muscle fibres, salted, spiced and dried in air for 10-14 days. Analysis per 100g: 11.5 g water, 1.9 g fat, 12.5 g ash, 65 protein, 308 kcal (1.3MJ).

Binary Fission. The method of reproduction of bacteria. The nucleic acids reproduce themselves and the cell divides into two daughter cells.

Biocytin. Refers to one of the bound forms of biotin which occurs naturally, the lysine derivative; not fully usable by all organisms until it has been hydrolysed to free biotin.

Bioflavonoids. Alternative name for flavonoids.

Biological Availability. The amount of a nutrient in a food is obtainable for use by the body. For example, the egg white protein avidin is able to bind the vitamin biotin making it completely biological unavailable; the essential amino acid lysine can undergo. Maillard reaction making such reacted lysines in a protein biologically unavailable.

Biological Oxygen Demand (BOD). A measure of microbial activity in a contaminated material. Used mainly to measure the potential for contamination as other methods give more accurate determination of microbial activity, e.g., colony counts.

Biological Value. Refers to a quantitative measure of the nutritive value of a protein food carried out under conditions where quality of the protein is the limiting factor. Defined as the amount of absorbed protein retained in the body (expressed as a ratio)-*i.e.*, digestibility is not taken into account. If digestibility is included (*i.e.* the amount retained is expressed as a fraction of the amount in the diet). The measure has been net protein utilisation. NPU = BV x digestibility. Previously it is expressed as a percentage scale, now as a ratio; thus the perfect protein has BA = 1.0 (100% retained), Examples are egg and human milk protein, 0.9-1.0; meat, fish and cow's milk, 0.75-0.8; wheat bread, 0.5; peanut, 0.44.45; gelatin, zero. When fed as mixers, these proteins complement one another.

Bios. Name given in 1901 by Wildiers to factor in cell-free extract of yeast necessary for growth of yea.. Later the precipitate was shown to be bios I (identified 1920 as inositol); and the filtrate, bios IIa,b beta-alanine, and IIb, biotin (isolated 1936).

Biostat. Trade name for ice having the antibiotic oxytetracycline.

Biosterol. Obsoleter name for vitamin A.

Biotin. Also termed as vitamin H, identical with bios II and with coenzyme R (growth factor and respiratory stimulant for the organism Rhizobium, present in the root nodules of legumes).

Essential to a wide variety of animals, including man, but synthesised in the intestines. It gets inactivated by combination with avidin, a protein in raw egg-white, and deficiency symptoms can be produced by feeding raw egg-while (not cooked). Deficiency causes dermatitis, loss of fur and disturbances of the nervous system in experimental animals. It occurs in liver kidney, off yolk yeast, vegetable, grains, nuts.

Biotoprotein. Refers to a soluble biotin protein compled that occurs naturally.

Birch Beer. Refers to non-alcoholic carbonated beverage which is flavoured with oil of wintergreen or oil of sweet birch and oil of sassafras.

Biscuit. Essentially a bakery confectionery dried down to low moisture content; name derived from Latin for twice-cooked. Obtained from soft flour: mostly rich in sugar and consequently of high energy content 420-510 kcal (1.7-2.1MJ) per 100g.

Termed cookie in the USA, where the word biscuit means

a small oake-like bun.

Biscuit Check. Refers to the development of splitting and cracks in bisuits immediately after banking.

Biskoids. Trade name for saccharine.

Bitot's Spots. Foam-like irregular plaques on the conjunctive of the eye, often seen in vitamin A deficiency but not considered to be a characteristic deficiency sign.

Bitters. Gentian, quassia and calumba, and in small doses, quinine and strychnine. Used to stimulate gustatory nerves in the mouth and thus stimulate appetite.

Biuret Test. For proteins (actually for peptide bonds). Violet colour gets developed when a drop of copper sulphate is added to a solution of protein in caustic soda.

Bixin. Carotenoid pigment which is found in the seeds of the tropical plant Bixa orellana: the crude extract is the colouring agent annatto, which see.

Blackberry. Berry of bramble, Rubus fructicosus. Analysis per 100g: protein 1.2g, fat 1.0g, 57 kcal (0.24 MJ), Fe 1.0 mg, vitamin A 50 g, vitamin B_1 0.03 mg, vitamin B_2 0.05 mg, nocotinic acid 0.4 mg, vitamin C 24 mg.

Black Currant. Fruit of the bush Ribes nigra. Of special interest as a fruit because of its high vitamin content. Analysis per 100 g: protein 0.9 g, fat trace carbohydrate 6.6g, water 77 g 29 kcal (0. 12MJ), Fe 1.3 mg, vitamin A 90g, vitamin B_1 0.03 mg. Vitamin B_2 0.06 mg, nicotinic acid 0.25 mg, vitamin C 200 mg.

Black Jack. Caramel.

Black PN. Food colour which it tetra sodium salt of 8-acetamido-2 (7-sulpho-4-*p*sulphophenyl-azo-1-naphthyazo) l-naphthol-3, 5-disulphonic acid. Also called Brilliant Black BN. Not very stable.

Black Tongue. Refers to a symptom of nicotinic acid deficiency in dogs, historically useful in the isolation of the vitamin.

Blaeberry. Bilberry.

Blanch. To part cook by dropping into hot water, (82-93°C), for 1-5 minutes. Fruit and vegetable are blanched before canning drying or freezing to soften their texture destroy enzymes, remove unpleasant flavours and air, or cause shrinkage. The destruction of enzymes in plant foods by denaturation through heating is important before freezing since without their destruction, they would continue to catalyse unwanted reactions at a slow rate and lower the quality of the food. Blanching can be used to remove unwanted salt or skins. It can cause the loss of 10-20% of sugars, salts, protein, niacin, some of the B vitamins and up to one third of the vitamin C.

Blanching. Blanch.

Blancmange Powders. Usually a cornflour base having added flavour and colour.

Bland Diet. One that is having the minimum of crude fibre or roughage and is therefore non-irritating and soothing to the intestine.

Blast Freezing. A method of freezing foods in which cooled air (–40° to –10°C) is blown around the food products by fans. Blast freezers are particularly useful for irregularly shaped foods which cannot be handled in a plate freezer.

Bleaching. In the context of food, this term usually refers to the bleaching of flour. Also refers to the bleaching of oils, a stage in the purification by which colloidally dispersed impurities and natural colouring matters are removed by activated earth or fuller's earth.

Bleaching Agents. Aging.

Bleeding Bread. Refers to a bacterial infection with Bacillus prodigious which stains the bread bright red. Under optimal conditions of warmth and damp the infection can appear overnight, and contamination of shewbread with this organism in churches - has led to accusations and riots against religious minorities over the centuries.

Blood Cells, White. Leucocytes.

Blood, Citrated. Blood that is prevented from clotting by the addition of citrate, which combines with the calcium. (Coagulation; blood) 600mg sodium citrate will prevent coagulation of 100ml blood.

Blood, Defibrinated. Blood clots rapidly after it is shed, when the soluble protein fibrinogen is converted into insoluble fibrin. If the blood gets stirred with a rod, the fibrin can be removed as it forms and the blood, still containing the cells, will remain fluid. This is defibrinated blood.

Blood, Oxalated. Blood that has been prevented from clotting by the addition of oxalate, which combines with the calcium. 160mg sodium oxalate will prevent the clotting of 100 ml blood.

Blood, Red Cells. Carry the red colouring matter, haemoglobin, which is the means of transporting oxygen and carbon dioxide in the blood stream. The cell, or erythrocyte, is 8.8 m in diameter, 1.9 m at its greatest thickness; 5 million per cubic millimetre of blood; exists for 120 days, then destroyed in the body, the iron being re-used.

Blood Sugar. The level of glucose in the blood which provides the energy for muscular metabolic and brain activity.

Blood Sugar Test. Glucose tolerance.

Blood Volume. Average males, 5.3*l*' females 3.8*l*; 78 and 66m*l* per kg body weight, respectively. Can be calculated from Wilson's formula : volume (ml) = 43 × weight (kg) + 131 × height (inches)-6250. Determined by injecting known amount of a dye, such as Evans Blue, and determining the degree of dilution in a sample of the blood.

Blood, White Cells. Leucocytes.

Bloom. Fat bloom has been the whitish appearance on the surface of chocolate which sometimes occurs on storage. It is due to a change in the form of the fat at the surface or to fat diffusing outward and being deposited on the surface.

Bloom Gelometer. An instrument which is used for measuring the strength of jellies, and also for any test of firmness, *e.g.*, staleness of bread.

For jelly strength the jelly is prepared at 6.66%

concentration and chilled at 10°C for 16-18 hours. The instrument measures the load in grams needed to produce a 4mm depression in the gel with a 1/2-inch diameter plunder. Gelatin at 250 Bloom grams finds use in jellied meat, at 200 in marshmallows.

Bloor Classification. A method of classifying lipids used by Bloor in 1926. He listed four classes:

1. simple lipids
2. compound lipids
3. glycolipids, and
4. the derived lipids.

Blueberry. High-bush blueberry (Vaccinium corymbosum) and low-bush (V. augustifolium) grown in North America.

Blue Cheese. Cheese, blue.

Blue Value.

1. Of vitamin A, this term refers to the transient blue colour produced by reaction with antimony trichloride, the depth of colour being proportional to the amount of the vitamin present.
2. Referring to starch, it has been an indeed of the free soluble starch, *i.e.*, the amylose, in a food, *e.g.*, potatoes.

Blue, VRS. Refers to sodium salt of 4,4' -di(diethylamino)-4",6" disulphotriphenylmethanolanhydride.

BMI. Body Mass Index.

BMR. Basal Metabolic Rate.

BOD. Biological Oxygen Demand.

Body-building Food. Term indiscriminately used, usually refers to proteins.

Body fluid. Water balance.

Body Mass Index. Weight (kg) divided by height (in) squared; used as index of obesity. It is same as Quetelet's index.

Body Surface. Surface area.

Bog Butter. Norsemen, Finns, Scots and Irish used to bury firkins of butter in bogs to ripen it for the strong flavour that developed.

(thea bohea) bu Roachelder, 1847, considered to be 'tannin'.

Boiled Sweets. Sugar and water boiled at such a high temperature, 149-166°C, that practically no water remains and a vitreous mass is formed on cooling. Actually a supersaturated solution of sugar.

Boil-in-the-bag. A food product is supplied par-cooked (partly cooked) -or raw in a plastic bag, normally made of high density polythene which can be cooked by immersing the bag in boiling water. Products which can be treated in this way are limited as such high temperature cooking often damages such food as meats and fish.

Bombay Duck. Fish occurring in Indian waters. These are eaten fresh or after salting and curing.

Bomb Calorimeter. Calorimeter.

Bone. Organic matrix of collagen, .osseoalbumoid and osseomucoid, with an inorganic mixture of 85% calcium phosphate, 10% calcium carbonate and 1.5% magnesium phosphate.

Bone Broth. Obtained by prolonged boiling of chopped bones. Of little nutrine value, having 2.4% gelatin, with very little calcium.

Bone Charcoal. Bones degreased, broken to required size and heated in closed retorts. The organic matter is carbonises, leaving about 10% carbon deposited on a framework of calcium phosphate. Used to purify solutions by virtue of its properties of absorbing colouring matter and impurities.

Bone Meal. Obtained from degreased animal bones and used as a supplement to both animal feed and human food as a source of both calcium and phosphate; also used as plant fertiliser as a source of phosphate.

Borage. A herb, Borage officinalis which is not grown on a commercial scale. The flowers and leaves are sometimes used to flavour beverages and have a flavour resembling that of cucumber.

Borax. Sodium salt of boric acid.

Boric Acid. Derived from boron; has in the past, been used as a food preservative (in bacon and margarine), but gets accumulated in the body.

Boston Brown Bread. In the United States, a spiced pudding steamed in the can.

Bottles. The customary wine bottle hold 700 to 750 ml. The two-bottle size is a magnum; four-bottle container is a Jecoboam; six is a Methusaleh; 12 is a Salamanzer: and 20 is a Nebuchadnezzar.

Botulism. Refers to the form of food poisoning which is caused by extremely potent neurotoxins of Clostridium botulinum (seven types of antigenically distinct todins have been identified). It is derived from botylus, a sausage, because the illness was originally associated with sausages in Germany.

Botulism has been rare but often fatal unless antitoxin gets administered, and arises from consumption of food that has been incorrectly preserved or treated and in which many of the competing micro-organisms have been destroyed. A wide range of foods have been involved, including meat, fish, milk, fruits and vegetable, and the toxin may be formed without any apparent spoilage of the food.

The toxin can be destroyed by heating at 80°C for ten minutes, but is more resistant in foodstuffs.

Bouillabaisse. Fish stew common in S.France. It is made from several kinds of fish and shellfish, cooked with oil, spices and herbs. So named since it is repeatedly boiled.

Bouillon. Plain, unclarified beef or veal broth.

Bottling. A similar process to canning but using glass bottles instead of cans *e.g.,* bottled milk.

Bound, Water. The water in a food which is bonded either strongly or weakly to other compounds but is not free water. Bound water cannot act as solvent for other compounds in the food and is not easily taken out by dehydration.

Bourbonal. Ethylvanillin; vanilla.

Bournvita. Trade name (Cadbury-Schweppes Ltd) for a

preparation of malt, milk, sugar, cocoa, eggs and flavouring, for consumption as a beverage when added to milk.

Analysis per 100g; protein 11.4g, fat 7.5g, carbohydrate 67.6g, Ca 89mg, Fe 3mg, kcal 370 (1.6 MJ).

Bovril. Trade name (Bovri Ltd) for a preparation of meat extract, hydrolysed beef, beef powder and yeast extract used as a beverage, breadspead and flavouring agent. Analysis per 100g: protein 28g, vitamin B_2 3.5mg, nicotinic acid 24mg, Fe 12mg.

Bowel. The lower end of the intestine joined to the ileum. Very little absorption of nutrients occurs in the bowel out it is here that water is taken up into the blood.

Bowman-Birk inhibitors. Refers to a group of protease inhibitors which are found, together with Kunits inhibitors, in soya beans.

Bradycardia. Refers to an unusually slow hear-beat; a symptom, among other causes, of certain vitamin deficiencies.

Bradyphagia. Eating very slowly.

Brain Sugar. One-time name for galactose.

Braise. Cook in a closed container with little liquid; usually in the oven.

Bran. Refers to the outer layers of cereal grain which are largely removed when the grain is milled-*i.e.*, in preparation of the white flour or white rice. The germ is discarded at the same time, and there occurs a considerable loss of iron and other minerals, and particularly of the B vitamins as well as of dietary fibre. Analysis of wheat bran per 100g has been as follows; 8g water, 4g sugars, 23g starch, 44g dietary fibre (mostly cellulose and hemicelluloses), 2.2g N (14g crude protein), 1.lg K, l.2g P, 13mg Fe, 16mg Zn, 0.9 mg thiamin, 0.4 mg riboflavin, 30mg niacin, 1.6mg vitamin E, 1.4mg vitamin B_6 Pv, 130g free folate, 2.4 mg pantothenate, 14g biotin.

Brandy. Refers to a spirit distilled from wine-name derived from German brantwein (burnt wine), corrupted to brandywine. 32% alcohol with only a trace of solids, 220 kcal (920kJ) per 100ml.

The age used to be designated by stars (one for 3 years old, two for 4, etc.) and initials VSO (very special old, 12-17 years), VSOP (very special old pale, 18-25 years), VVSOP (very, very special old pale, up to 40 years old), but these have largely lost their meaning through indiscriminate usage.

Brawn. Produced from meat, ears and tongue of the pig; boiled with peppercorns and herbs, minced and pressed into a mould. Mock brawn differs in that other meat by-products are used.

Bread. Usually refers to a loaf which is made from wheat or rye flour, but mixtures of ninny cereals may be used. Wheat flour makes a softer loaf than other cereals, because the gluten is extensible and holds pockets of air. White bread is extensible and holds pockets of air. White bread is generally made from flour of 72% extraction rate, the composition depends on the type of flour used.

Analysis per 100g wholemeal bread (unenriched white bread of 72% extraction rate) the composition depends on the type of flour used.

Analysis per 100g wholemeal bread (unenriched white bread of 72% extraction flour shown in parentheses): 40g water (39), 8.8g protein (7.8), 2.7g fat (1.7), 38g carbohydrate (45), 2.5 rug Fe (1.3), 2mg Zn (0.8), 8.5g dietary fibre (2.7), 26 mg thiamin (0.06), 0.06 mg riboflavin (0.03), 3.9 mg niacin-largely unavailable (0.5), 22 g free folate (6), 0.6mg pantothenate (0.3), 6 g biotin (1), 360 mg phytic acid (4), 216 kcal or 0.22 MJ (233 kcal or 0.92 MJ).

Brown breads are obtained from flours of varying extraction rates between wholemeal and white flours. Added nutrients are present in, for example, protein bread, wheat germ bread, gluten bread and milk bread.

Bread, Acerated. The dough is made with water saturated with carbon dioxide under pressure. The main aim is to produce an aerated loaf without the loss of carbohydrate involved in a yeast fermentation (7% of the total ingredients). The result was insipid in flavour and the method went out of use.

Bread, Black. Coarse wholemeal wheat or rve bread leavened with sauertag *i.e.,* mixture of fermenting micro-organisms. These includes:

1. Peptonising bacteria that turn the dough to a more plastic state.
2. Yeast.
3. Lactic or acetic bacteria that produce the sour flavour.

Bread Brown. A loaf may not legally be described as brown (or wholemeal) unless it contains not less than 0.6% fibre (on dry weight) i.e., a high rate of extraction.

Bread. Cornell. Loaf increased nutritional value by adding 6% soya flour and 8% skin milk solids. So called due to participation of staff of Cornell university in its development.

Breadfruit. Refers to the starchy fruit of the tree Artocarpus communis or A. incia. Staple though seasonal food of the West Indies; eaten roasted whole when ripe or boiled in pieces when green.

Analysis per 100g; water 70g, carbohydrate 26g, protein 1.5g, fat 0.4. kcal 113 (0.47 MJ), Fe 1mg, vitamin B_1 0.06 mg, nicotinic acid 1.2mg, vitamin C 20 mg.

Bread, lactein. Loaf with added milk, usually about 6% milk solids, although 3-4% milk solids are often added to the ordinary loaf in the United States.

Bread, Soda. Bread which is leavened with sodium bicarbonate and an acidic substance instead of yeast, although legally it may contain yeast as well.

Bread, Starch-reduced. Bread is usually 9-10% protein and about 50% starch; if the starch is reduced either by washing some part of it out of the dough or by adding extra protein, the bread is termed as starch-reduced, and is generally claimed of value in slimming and diabetic diets.

Legally the term 'starch-reduced bread' may be applied

only to bread containing less then 50% carbohydrate and the wording claiming its value as a slimming aid is legally controlled.

Breakfast Food, Cereal. May be defined as any food obtained by the swelling, roasting, grinding, rolling or glaking or any cereal. Described under individual names (*e.g.*, All-bran; Bemax; Cornflakes; Wheat, puffed; Wheat shredded; Force)

Brewers' Grains. General residue from brewing, having about 25% protein: used as animal feed, and also a source of unidentified growth factors.

Brewer, Pounds. Before specific gravity was used in breweries, the strength of wort was expressed as the difference between the weight of a barrel of wort and that of a barrel of water (360 lb). The excess weight over 360 lb is represented by brewers' pounds.

Brewing. Beer.

Brine. A solution containing about 25% sodium chloric (NaCl), 1% potassium nitrate (KNO_2) and 0.1% sodium nitrate ($NaNO_2$), used for curing meats and in canning some vegetables.

Brislings. Young sprats, Culpea sprattus. Canned brislings are having 300 g vitamin A and 2550 g vitamin D per 100 g.

Brix. Refers to a table of specific gravity which is based on the Balling tables and is calculated in grams of cane sugar in 100 g solution at 20°C, *i.e.* degree Brix = percentage sugar. Used to refer to concentration of sugar syrups used in canned fruits.

Broil. US term for girl.

Broiler Chicken. Chicken.

Bromatology. Refers to science of foods (from the Greek broma, food).

Bromelains. Refers to proteolytic enzymes in pineapple (Ananas comosus) and related members of Bromelidaceae; available as by products from commercial pineapple production, usually from the stems: similar in activity to ficin (from the fig) and papain (from pawpaw), and used to tenderise meat, to treat sausage casings and to chill-proof beer.

Brominated Oils. Brominated olive, peach, apricot kernel, soya oils, etc. It is used to help to stabilise emulsions of flavouring substances in softs drinks; also described as weighting oils. In India, these are banned because they are careinogenic.

Brose. Scottish dish which is obtained by pouring boiling water on oatmeal or barely meal; fish meat or vegetables may be added.

Broth. Soup made from meat or bone extractives, with vegetables, meat, farinaceous material, spices and herbs.

Brown Colours Brown *FK.* A mixture of the disodium salt of 1.3-diamino-4,6-di(*p*sulphophenylazo) benzene and the sodium salt of 2,4-diamino-5-(*p*-sulphophenylazo) toluene- 'kipper brown'.

Chocolate- Brown FB. The product of coupling diazotised naphthionic acid with a mixture of morin and maclurin.

Chocolate Brown HT. Disodium salt of 2,4-dihydroxy-3, 5di(sulphor-l-naphthylazo) benzyl alcohol. Both these colours have been 'baking browns'.

Browning Reaction. Maillard reaction; phenol oxidases.

Brussels Sprouts. Leaf buds of Brassica Oleracea Gemmifera.

Analysis per 100g; protein 3.6 g, fat 0.4 g, Ca 26mg, Fe 1.0mg, kcal 36 (0.15 MJ), vitamin A 90 g, vitamin B_1 0.06mg, vitamin B_2 0.12mg, nicotinic acid 0.5mg, vitamin C 70 mg.

Buckling. Hot-smoked herring. (The kipper is cold-smoked.)

Buckwheat. Refers to a cereal, Fagopyrum esuculentum. It is also known as saracen corn and, when cooked, as the cooked grain, porridge or pancakes.

Analysis per 100g; protein 11g, fat 2g, carbohydrate 70g; kcal 350 (1.5 Mi), Fe 3mg, vitamin B_1 0.3mg, vitamin B_Z 0.3mg nicotinic acid 3mg.

Budde's Process. For preserving milk.

Budding. A process in yeast and some other organisms where a new individual is produced by part of the mother cell or individual growing out into a bud. The bud is eventually pinched off as a new organism.

Buffers. Refers to which are substances that resist change in acidity or alkalinity. Salts of weak acids and weak bases are buffers, also proteins and amino acids by virtue of their content of both acidic and basic groups.

Bulb. An organ in some plants which consists of a underground axis with many thick overlapping leaves, for example, onions and garlic.

Bulgur. Prepared, precooked wheat originating in the Near East. Wheat is soaked cooked and dried; it is lightly milled to remove the outer bran and cracked. Eaten with soups ,cooked with meat etc.

Bulgur has been the oldest processed food known; also called ala and American rice; cooked with meat it is called kibbe.

Bullace. Wild damson.

Burghul. Alternative name for bulgur.

Bring Feet Syndrome. Aching and throbbing in the feet which is later spreading upwards to the knees. It results from long periods on a diet which is poor in protein and B vitamins.

Claimed to be cured by pantothenic acid but no confirmed and the whole vitamin B complex appears to be necessary.

Bushel. Refers to the measure of capacity. It is equivalent to 80lb of distilled water at 17°C with barometer reading 30 inches, *i.e.* 8 gallons or 4 pecks. Used as a measure of corn, potatoes etc.

The weight of a bushel varies with the product-e.g. Wheat 60lb; maize 56lb; rye 56lb; barley 48lb; oats 32lb; paddy rice 45lb.

The American measure has been the Winchester bushel, which is 3% greater.

Butane Diol (Butylene Glycol). $CH_3CHOHCHOHCH_3$. Colourless liquid. It is soluble in both water and ether, having an energy content of 6 kcal (24 kJ) per g.

Butanedione. A chemical in butter formed by bacteria

which gives the characteristic butter smell and flavour. Butanedione is added to margarine give it the flavour of butter. More commonly known as directly.

Butt. Cash for beer or wine having 108 imperial gallons.

Butter. Obtained from milk fat by souring the cream either naturally or with a bacterial culture (starter) followed by churning. Usually not less than 80% fat, the remainder being water; 2% salt sometimes added; contains trace of protein and lactose; 740 kcal (3MJ) per 100g; may be coloured with annatto. Vitamin A about 1000 g per 100g, partly as carotene, higher on summer than winter; vitamin D 0.6-1.0 g, vitamin E 2 g.

Butter, Black. Butter which is browned by heating, vinegar, salt, pepper or other seasoning then being added, and finds use as a sauce.

Butterine. Margarine.

Buttermilk. Residue which is left after churning butter, 0.1- 0.20% fat with the other milk constituent proportionately increased. Having a slightly acid flavour together with a distinctive flavour due to diacetyl and related substances.

Buttermilk, Cultured. Refers to the modern equivalent of sour buttermilk, produced by acid-producing streptococci in skim milk.

Butter, Process or Renovated. Butter that has been melted and rechurned with the addition of milk, cream or water.

Butter Vegetable. Vegetable butters.

Butter, Whey (serum butter). Obtained from the small amount of fat left in whey. It has a fatty acid composition slightly different from that of ordinary butter.

Butylated Hydroxyanisole (BHA). An antioxidant which is used for fats and fatty foods, derived chemically from phenol, not destroyed by heat and therefore useful in baked products; active at concentration of 0.01-0.1%.

Butylated Hydroxytoluene(BHT). Antioxidant which is used for fats and fatty foods.

Butyric acid. $CH_3CH_2CH_2COOH$. A short chain fatty acid found in triglycerides of butter and making up about 5-6% of their weight. Small amounts are also found in other fats.

Butyrine. Alternative name for alpha-amino-n-butyric acid. It occurs in the blood stream, derived from threonine and not present in the diet.

BV. Biological value.

Bynin. Name assigned (by Osborne and Campbell, 1896) to an alcohol-soluble protein of malt; later shown to be identical with the alcohol soluble protein of barley, and the name was abandoned.

C

Cadaverine. 1-5-pentanediamine. It is formed by decarboxylation of lysine, and found in decomposting meat and fish; toxic.

Cadmium. This mineral gets accumulated in the body throughout life, reaching 20-30 mg (200-300 mol), but does not appear to be a dietary essential. Cadmium poisoning is a recognised industrial hazard. In Japan it has been incriminated in itai-itai disease, a severe and sometimes fatal loss of calcium from bone tissue—the disease taken place in an— area where rice was grown on land irrigated with contaminated waste waters. Experimentally, the toxic effects of small doses of cadmium could be reversed with zinc (possibly owing to competition).

Caecum. Refers to first part of the large intestine, separated from the small intestine by the ileo-colic sphincter. It is small in carnivorous animals, very large herbivores as it gets involved in cellulose digestion, of intermediate size in man.

Caffeine. Alkaloid drug (trimethylxanthine) occurring in coffee and tea. Raises blood pressure, stimulates kidneys and averts fatigue temporarily.

Coffee beans have 1 % caffeine; hence the beverage contains about 18mg per oz or 100mg per cup. Tea contains 1.5-2.5% caffeine, about 12-15mg per oz of beverage. Coladrinks contain 3-4.5 mg per oz

Also called theine.

Caffeol. Volatile oil which gives characteristic flavour and aroma to coffee.

Calamodin. A citrus fruit which is resembling a small tangerine, having a delicated pulp and a lime-like flavour.

Calcium. A mineral present in milk products, fish , hard water and in bread, which is required for healthy bones and teeth, to aid in the clotting of blood and in muscles. The average adult human requires 1.1 grams per day and the total body content is about 1000 grams.

Calcium Acid Phosphate. Also known as monocalcium phosphate, and acid calcium phosphate or ACP, $Ca(H_4PO_4)_2$. It finds use as the acid ingredient of baking powder and self-raising flour since it reacts with bicarbonate to liberate carbon dioxide.

Chemically it is similar to "superphosphate' fertiliser but purer.

Calcium Activated Neutral Proteinase (CANP). A proteolytic enzyme-found in meat which breaks down the contracted muscle proteins during conditioning.

Calcium Gluconate. Water-soluble salt of calcium and gluconic acid which is useful for intravenous administration (*e.g.* in the relief of tetany).

Calcium-Phosphate Ratio. Rickets can be caused in the rat by feeding diet with a high ratio of calcium to phosphate, and it was thought at one time that the ratio for man should lie between 1:2 and 2:1, but within the range normally ingested phosphate does not appear to have any effect on the absorption of calcium, except possibly in young infants.

Calculus. A stone which gets formed in tissue like kidney and gall bladder. Kidney stones consist of uric acid, urates, and calcium oxalate, carbonate and phosphate. Possibly of dietary causation.

Renal calculus—stones in kidney or ureter.

Vesical calculus—prostatic gland obstruction.

Biliary calculus—gallstone, which see.

Calorie. The unit of heat used in nutrition has been the kilocalorie, amount of heat required to raise the temperature of 1kg of water from 15°C to 16°C, abbreviated to kcal or written with a capital C to distinguish it from the small calorie.

Calories, Empty. Refers to foods that supply only energy with little, if any, of the nutrients.

Calorie Values. Energy.

Calorimeter (bomb calorimeter). An instrument which is used for measuring the amount of oxidisable energy present in a substance by burning it in oxygen and measuring the heat released. The heat liberated by burning a food in this way will coincide with the metabolisable energy in that food only if it can be completely metabolished. For example, proteins liberate 5.65 kcal/g in the bomb calorimeter in which the nitrogen is oxidised to the dioxide, but only 4.4 kcal/g in the body where the nitrogen gets excreted as urea and uric acid, etc. (Containing 1.25 kcal/g)

Calvin Cycle. Carbon fixation in plants.

Camphell's Process. A method of drying milk by first concentrating by blowing hot air through, followed by drum-drying.

Campden Process. Refers to the preservation of food by the addition of sodium bisulphite, which liberates sulphur dioxide. Also known as cold preservation, since it replaces heat sterilisation.

Campden Tablets. Tablets of sodium bisulphite.

Camu-Camu. A peruvian fruit from the bush Myrciaria parensis; burgundy red in colour, 6-14g weight, 3cm diameter: 3000mg vitamin C per 100g pulp.

Can. A metal container used for canning which can be sealed to prevent contamination by micro-organisms.

Canapes. Small open sandwiches.

Canbra Oil. Oil extracted from genetically selected variety of rape-seed with not more than 2% erucic acid.

Cancer. The second most common cause of early death in the Western world . Cancer is a groups of diseases in which cells reproduce themselves out of control. It has been linked with dietary patterns in recent years.

Candiet Peel. Used in confectionery. It is prepared by softening the peel, often of citrus fruits, and boiling for prolonged period with sugar syrup.

Candy.

1. Crystallised sugar which is made by repeated boiling and slow evaporation.
2. United States term for sugar confectionery.

Candy Docter. Sugar doctor.

Cane Sugar. Refers to sucrose which is extracted from the sugar cane; identical with sucrose prepared from any other source, such as sugar beet.

Canner's Alkali. Mixture of sodium hydroxide and sodium carbonate which is used to remove skin from fruit before canning (sodium-hydroxide alone more frequently used).

Canning, Aseptic. Foods can be pre-sterilised at very high temperatures, 150-175°C, for a few seconds and then sealed into cans under aseptic conditions. The flavour, colour and vitamin retention have been superior with this short time, high temperature process compared with conventional canning.

The rate of bacterial spore destructions has been approximately multi tenfold for very 10°C rise in temperature, while the chemical reactions responsible for loss of quality get doubled for every 10°C rise in temperature.

Canthaxanthin. Refers to a red carotenoid pigment which is chemically related to beta-carotene but without any vitamin A activity. Suggested use as addition to the diet of broiler chickens to impart a pigmented skin and shanks, and to the diet of trout to produce the bright colours of wild trout; these colours are normally derived from natural foodstuffs, which may be variable or in short supply.

Similarly, beta apo-8-carotenal, which has been four-fifths of the beta-carotene molecule, can be used in chick diets to increase the colour of the egg yolks.

Capers. Buds of unopened flowers of Capparis spinosa

flavour for pickles and sauces.

Capillary Fragility. Refers to the resistance to rupture of the walls of a blood vessel, which would result in the leakage of red blood cells into the tissue spaces.

Capon. Castrated cockerel; slightly increased growth with more tender flesh than the cockerel. Surgery mostly replaced by 'chemical caponisation', *i.e.* implantation of pellets of female sex hormone.

Capric Acid. A fatty acid, $C_9H_{19}COOH$. Occurs as triglyceride in coconut, in goat and cow butter and in the fat of the spice bush.

Caproic Acid. A fatty acid, $C_6H_{11}COOH$. Found as triglyceride in goat and cow butter and coconut oil and human fat.

Caprylic Acid. A fatty acid, $C_7H_{15}COOH$. Occurs as triglyceride in goat and cow butter, coconut oil and human fat.

Capsicum. Pepper.

Caramel. Brown substance which is made when carbohydrates especially sugars are heated in solution. Caramel is used to colour and flavour many foods *e.g.* beer sauces.

Caramels. Toffee.

Caramelization. The reaction of sugars with each other when they are heated, especially when there is no water present. Caramilization results in the formation of brown substances with a characteristic flavour.

Caraway. Refers to the dried ripe fruit of Carum carvi. Main component of the volatile oil is carvone, with smaller amounts of limonene. Used for the liquer kummel, and on bread and rolls.

Carbohydrate by Difference. In the analysis of foods it has been difficult to determine the various carbohydrates and they have been usually approximated by subtracting the measured protein plus ash plus fat from total. The figure can be corrected by subtracting dietary fibre which is non-available carbohydrate.

Carbohydrate by difference has been the sum of:

(a) unavailable carbohydrate–pentosans, pectins, hemicelluloses and celluloses;
(b) available carbohydrate—dextrins, starch and sugars;
(c) non-carbohydrates, such as organic acids and lignin.

Carbohydrate Metabolism. Glucose metabolism.

Carbohydrates. Substances that are composed of carbon, hydrogen and oxygen with two atoms of hydrogen for every oxygen. They include polysaccharides like starch, dextrins and glycogen which are digested to glucose, and sugars such as lactose, fructose and glucose, as well as undigestible materials.

They form the major part of the diet of man in the form of starch and sucrose in particular, and provide energy at the rate of 4 kcal or 16 kJ per g. The loss of water in the formation of disaccharides and polysaccharides from the monosaccharides causes slight differences in energy content-monosaccharides 3.75 kcal or 15.6 kJ, diaccharides 3.95 kcal or 16.5kJ, starch 4.18 kcal or 17.5 kJ and glycerol 4.32 kcal or 18.0 kJ per g.

Carbohydrates, Unavailable. The term includes pentosans, pectins, hemicellulose, cellulose, lignin and gums which are not digested and therefore unavailable to monogastric animals, but some have been available to ruminants.

Carbon Dioxide, Available. Baking powder; flour, self-raising.

Carbon dioxide Storage. Gas storage.

Carbonic Anhydrase. Enzyme that is able to convert carbon dioxide and water into carbonic acid. It is normally a slow process and its acceleration by the enzyme is an essential part of respiration (transfer of carbon dioxide from the tissues to the lungs). Present in red blood cells; plays part in gastric secretion of hydrochloric acid; contains zinc.

Carboxymethylccellulose. Produced from the pure cellulose of cotton or wood. Absorbes up to 50 times its weight of water to form a stable colloidal mass, and used in combination with stabilisers as a whipping agent, (in ice-cream, confectionery, jellies, etc,) and as an inert food filler in slimming aids.

Carboxypeptidase. Refers to an enzyme of the pancreatic juice which splits polypeptides to dipeptides. Removes the terminal unit of the chain in which the carboxyl radical is free; hence, it is an exopeptidase.

Carcinogen. A substance which is able to induce cancer.

Cardamom. Dried, nearly ripe, fruit, and the seed of Elettatia car-damomum (ginger family). The volatile oil is having cineol and terpineol. It finds use as flavouring in sausages, in bakery goods and in cury powder, and used in whole, mixed pickling spice.

Carmine-fibrin. Chopped blood fibrin that is soaked in ammoniacal carine solution. It finds use as a test of proteolytic activity since, when digestion takes place, the liberation of the carmine into the solution acts as an indicator.

Carminic Acid. An aromatic compound containing three rings of carbon atoms found in cochineal. When carminic acid reacts with aluminium (Al) it forms a lake called carmine.

Carmoisine. Red colour permitted in food in many other countries. It is also called Azorubin; disodium salt of 2-(4-sulpho-1- naphthylazo)-1-naphthol-4-sulphonic acid.

Carnitine. Plays a role in transferring the acetyl group from inside the mitochondroin to the outside, where fat synthesis occurs (Y-Trimethy-Y-Hydroxybutyrobetaine). It is found in animal muscle, and is particularly rich in meat extract but is not a dietary essential for man and the higher animals. The only organisms that have been shown to require carnitine as a dietary essential are the mealworm and a few related species. It was originally called vitamin B_1.

Carnosine. Beta-adnyl histidine. A dipeptide which is found in muscle of most animals; function unknown.

Carob Seed. Seeds and pod of Ceratonia siliqua, also known as locust bean and St. John's bread. Contains a sweet pulp which is rich in sugar and gums; used for fodder and for the preparation of carob-seed gum used for emulsifier, cosmetics and textile sizes.

Carotenal. (β-apo-8'-carotenal). Red-orange carotenoid pigment. It is used as a food colour in many countries; has vitamin A activity.

Carotene. Red pigment in plants; obvious in carrots, red palm oil and yellow maize, masked by chlorophyll in leaves.

It gets converted into retinol in the body. About one-third of the vitamin A of diets has been supplied as carotene. Present to only a limited extent in animal tissues: for example, there is some carotene as well as tetnol in milk. It occurs in three forms-α—, β— and γ-carotenes -and lends name to a range of pigments of similar structure, the carotenoids, only a few of which are vitamin A-active.

It is used as a colouring materials in foods and as a source of vitamin A in vegetarian and kosher margarines.

Carotenoids. A group of red, yellow and orange pigments found in most plants. They are not synthesized by animals and so must be taken in the diet. Carotenoids are used by humans to make vitamin A.

Carotenols. Carotenoid pigments carrying the hydroxyl group.

Caroto—albumin. Carotene-protein compled in the blood serum. It is made of transport of carotene in the body.

Carrageenan. A mixture of two polysaccharide hydrocolloids which contains sulphate and can be extracted from seaweed.

Carrot. Root of Daucus carota which is commonly used as a vegetable; an extremely rich source of carotene-5-15 mg per 100g. The lower range occurs in the young carrots harvested in early summer, higher values in the older carrots.

Analysis per 100 g: water 90 g, sugar 5g, protein 0.7-0.9g, 20 kcal 90 kJ).

Car-price Reaction. Test for vitamin A which gives a blue colour with a solution of antimony trichloride in chloroform (the Carprice reagent).

Cater's Spread. Name assigned to a mixture of butter (68%) with hydrigenated oil (12.4%) plus salts, preservative and lecithin, used as a breadspread.

Cartilage. Consists mainly of collagen, chondromucoid (protein plus chondroitin sulphuric acid) and chondroalbumoid (a protein similar to elastin). New bone growth consists of cartilage on which calcium salts are deposited at a later stage to form the bone.

Carton. A container, usually made from plastic or cardboard, in which foods are stored e.g., milk.

Case Hardening. The process by which small molecules, such as salts and sugars gather at the surface of foods during dehydration and form a skin.

Casein. The main protein of milk it accounts for nearly 80% of all the protein in milk. Casein is a mixture of several proteins which combine together in milk to form micelles with calcium phosphate.

Casein, lodinated (caseoiodine). Casein with about 9% iodine introduced into the molecule; has some thyroactive properties similar to those of thyroxine.

Caseoiodine. Iodinated casein having about 90% iodine.

Cassareep. Refers to the juice of the bitter cassva or manioc. It is boiled to a thick syrup and used as a base for sauces.

Cassava. (manioc). Tuber of the plant Manihot utilissima. Staple article of diet in many tropical countries, although an extremely poor source of protein.

Analysis per 100 g: protein 0.9 g. fat 0.2 g, Ca 25 mg, Fe 0.5 mg, kcal 109 (0.46 MJ), vitamin B_1 0.04 mg, vitamin B_2 0.02 mg, nicotinic acid 0.4 mg, vitamin C 27 mg.

The juice from the roots is cassareep which is used in sauces and fermented with molasses. The leaves are eaten as a vegetable. The tuber is a source of tapioca.

Cassia. Refers to the inner bark of a tree grown in the Far East-used as a seasoning; similarly in appearance and flavour to cinnamon.

Cassia. Beverage (tea substitute) which is made from curd leaves of holly bush, Ilex cassine; contains 1-1.6%

caffeine and 8% tannin.

Castor Oil. From the castor oil bean, Ricinus. The oil itself is non-irritating, but in the small intestine it gets hydrolysed by lipase to liberate ricinoleic acid, which is an irritant to the gastrointestinal mucosa and therefore acts as a purgative.

Catabolism. The breakdown of food molecules inside the cell to produce energy and the compounds used in synthesis.

Catalase. Enzyme in plants and animals which splits hydrogen peroxide into water and gaseous oxygen. It is a conjugated protein having haem (identical with the haem of haemoglobin) as its prosthetic group.

Catalysis. The process by which a catalyst speeds up a chemical reaction.

Catalyst. Substance that alters the rate of a chemical reaction; mostly of use when it accelerates the reaction. Enzymes are defined as organic catalysts produced by living cells. Catchup. Alternative spelling of catsup or ketchup.

Catechol. A phenolic compound consisting of a benzene ring and two hydroxyl (-OH) functional groups commonly found in fruit, particularly apples. Catechol is an important example of the diphenolic substances of the polyphenolases which cause enzymic browing.

Cathepsins. Group of intracellular proteolytic enzymes in animal tissues. There are four enzymes in the group, cathepsins I, II, III and IV, respectively similar to pepsin, trypsin, aminopeptidase and car boxypeptidase.

Tomato ketchup.

Cauliflower. Refers to white edible flower of Brassica oleracea botrytis. Horticulturally, varieties that mature in summer and autumn are cauliflowers and those that mature in winter are broccoli, but commonly both are called cauliflower.

Analysis per 100g raw: 93 g water, 1.5 g sugars, 2.1 g dietary fibre. 1.9 g protein, 13 kcal (55kJ), 0.1 mg thiamin, 0.1 mg riboflavin, 0.6 mg niacin, 50-90 mg vitamin (2,0.2 mg free folate, 0.6mg pantothenate, trace carotene).

Causative Agent. A chemical, micro-organism or other factor which is responsible for food poisoning.

Caciar(e). Salted hard roe of the sturgeon (Acipenseridae family). Analysis per 100g:30g protein, 20g fat, nil carbohydrate, 340kcal (1.42 MJ).

Celeriac. Turnip-rooted celery, Apium graveolens var. rapaceum, of which the swollen base of the steam has been the edible part; closely related to celery but the stems are small and bitter.

Analysis per 100g, boiled: 90g water, 2g carbohydrate, 4.9g dietary fibre, 1.6g protein, 14kcal (60kJ), traces of B vitamins, about 4mg vitamin C.

Celery. Edible stems of Apium graveolens.

Analysis per 100g, raw : 93.5g water, 1.3g carbohydrate, 1.8g dietary fibre, 0.9g protein, 8kcal (36kJ), trace of B vitamins, approximately 7mg vitamin C.

Celiac Diseace. Coeliac disease.

Cell Membrane. The double membrane surrounding the contents of the cell.

Cellobiose. Two molecules of glucose which are joined together in the 1,4'—β position (as distinct from the 1,4'—α bond in maltose). Cellobiose is the basic structural unit of cellulose.

Celluflour. Powdered cellulose. It finds use in experimental diets to provide indigestible bulk.

Cellulase. Enzyme that attacks cellulose. It is present in the digestive juices of various snails, wood—boring insects, and microorganisms. The cellulase present in the intestinal micro—organisms of ruminants is responsible for the ability of these animals to get energy from straw, for their own degestive juices do not contain cellulase.

Cellulose. A polysaccharide that forms the supporting cell structure in plants; does not occur in animals. Having long chain of glucose units.

It is not digested in man or other monogastric animals,

but serves a useful purpose in providing bulk for intestinal functioning. It is digested by the bacteria in the rumen of ruminating animals, which can therefore subsist on grass and hay.

In the native state molecular weight is 600 000-15 million.

Alpha-cellulose is having m.wt 80 000-340 000. Acid hydrolysis is able to convert this into microcrystallune cellulose, m.wt 30 000—50 000, used as filler in 'slimming foods'.

Centrifugation. A process by which liquid samples are spun around at high speed to cause the accelerated settling of particles in suspension.

Centrifuge. Machine that exerts a pull many times stronger than gravity by spinning. It is used to clarify liquids by settling the heavier solid in a few minutes, a process that might take several days under gravity. Also used to separate two liquids of different densities-e.g., cream from milk.

Cereal Coffee. Prepared from roasted cereal grains.

Cereals. The term used for any grain or edible fruit of the grass family which may be used as food. Include wheat, rice, oats, rye, barley, maize and millet.

Cerebrose. One time name for galactose.

Cerebrosides. Refer to the part of the structural matter of brain and the myelin sheath of nerves. It is having phrenosin, kerasin, fatty acid, sphingosine and galactose. This is the only structure of the body that contains the sugar galactose.

Cerelose. Commercial glucose having about 9% water.

Ceruloplasmin. Copper-protein complex which constitutes major part of circulating blood copper in man (and other mammals). It is involved in iron metabolism.

Cetavlon. Trade name ICI for detergent and bacteriostat, cetyltrimethylammonium bromide.

Cetyl Alcohol. Solid, waxy, straight—chain alcohol of sixteen carbon atoms. It occurs in spermaceti (from the sperm whale) and waxes.

Can be spread as a thin (monomolecular) film on the surface of water in reservoirs, where it reduces evaporation of the water.

CF. Citrovorum Factor.

Chalazae. The fibrous protein structures of the egg white which hold the yolk in place.

Chalva. Halva.

Chamomile. Can be either of two herbs, Anthemis nobilis and Mactricaria recutica. An essential oil which is used for flavouring liqueurs; chamomile tea, made by infusing dried flower heads, used as old—fashioned tonic; whole herb used to make herb yolk beers.

Chapati (chapati or chuppati). Flat, unleavened Indian bread which is made from wheat flour or miller.

Charcoal. Bone charcoal.

Charqui. Refers to the dried meat of Brazil, chiefly from beer but also from sheep, llama and alpaca in Peru. Strips of meat cut lengthways and pressed after salting, then air—dried; finished form is in flat, thin sheets, rather flacky, so differing from the long strips of biltong.

Chartreuse. Liqueur which was originally made by monks of Chartreux, using, it is said, more than 200 ingredients. There are three varieties : green 96% of proof spirit; yellow, 74.5%; and white 52.5%.

Chastek Paralysis. Refers to acute dietary disease of foxes which is caused by the inclusion of 10% of raw fish in the diet. It is due to a deficiency of vitamin B_1 caused by the presence of the enzyme thaiaminase in the fish, which destroys the vitamin. It is cured by adding vitamin B_1 to the diet.

CHD. Coronary heart disease.

Cheddaring. In the manufacture of cheese, after coagulation of the milk, heating of the curd and draining, the curds are piled along the floor of the vat, when, in the case of Cheddar cheese, they consolidate to a rubbery sheet of curd. This stage is called the cheddaring process. (Cheshire cheese is not allowed to settle so densely and has a more crumbly texture).

Cheese. A fresh or aged product made by coagulating milk, cream, skin milk concentrated milk, buttermilk, dried milk or any combi-nation of these with rennet. The solids, called the curd are sepa-rated from the liquid left after coagulation, called whey and are pressed to a firm cake to form the cheese. Most cheeses are fermented with bacterial cultures over a period of time before being eaten. There are more than 400 known varieties of cheese in the world.

Cheese, Blue. Cheese that is having an internal growth of the mould peni cillium ropueforti-e.g., Blue Vinney, Stilton and Roque—fort.

Cheese, Cottage (Pot cheese, Dutch cheese, Schmierkase). Refers to soft, uncured white cheese made from pasteurised skin milk (or milk powder) by lactic acid starter with or without added rennet), heated, washed and drained (salt may be added). Having more than 80% water.

Farm cheese is as above but the curd is pressed.

Cheese, Processed. Natural cheese passes its peak of flavour rapidly and processing temporarily arrests the deterioration. Processed cheese is loaf cheese, melted, pasteurised, with flavouring added (Pimento, caraway, etc.), plus emulsifiers, and repacked.

Nutritive value identical with that of original cheese.

Cheese, Whey. Prepared from whey by heat—coagulation of the proteins (lactalbumin and lactoglobulin).

Chelating Agents. Refers to the substances that react with metal ions and remove them from their sphere of action; hence, also called sequestrants. These are used to-remove traces of metals which may cause food to deteriorate, clinically to reduce absorption of a mineral, in garden soils, and in chemical operations.

Chemical Food Poisoning. The food poisoning caused by harmful chemicals present in food, e.g., oxalic acid in rhubarb leaves, plant lectins. Some harmful chemicals in food may result from their use by man, e.g., compounds may be used to protect food cops during growth but, if still present at harvest can cause a risk of food poisoning.

Chemical Ice. Ice having chemicals used as preservative- e.g., a solution of antibiotics or other chemicals frozen and used to preserve fish.

Chemical Score. Chemical method of defining the nutritional value of proteins, proposed by Block and Mitchell (1946). The limiting amino acid in the protein under consideration is expressed as the percentage of the same amino acid present in egg taken as the standard. Chemical score numerically equals biological value.

A later modification has been protein score, in which a standard acid reference mixture is used instead of off protein.

Chemotheraphy. Means the treatment of diseaseby chemicals that have toxic effect on the micro—organisms.

Cherry. Fruit of Prunus species.

Analysis per 100g : protein 1.0g. fat 0.4g. kcal 54 (0.23 MJ), Fe 0.4 mg, carotene 170 g vitamin B_1 0.05 mg, vitamin B_2 0.05 mg, nicotinic acid 0.4 mg, vitamin C 7mg.

Cherry, West Indian. Fruit of a small bushy tree native to tropical and semi-tropical regions of America- Malpighia punicifolia. The richest known source of vitamin C; the edible portion of the fruit has 1000mg of vitamin C per 100g when ripe, and the green fruit 3000mg. Also known as Barbados cherry and acerola (Spanish), and Antilles cherry.

Chervil.

1. A herb, Anthriscus cerefolium, with parsley—like leaves, it is used in the fresh green state as a garnish and for flavouring salads and soups.

2. Turnip rooted chervil, Chaerophyllum, bulbosum a hardly, bienial vegetable cultivated for its roots.

Chestnut, Water. Trapa natans, also know as caltrops and singharanut. Seed is eaten raw or roasted.

Analysis per 100g: 3g protein, 15g carbohydrate, 75 kcal (0.32 MJ), 0.8 mg iron, 0.05 mg vitamin B_1 0.06 mg nicotinic acid, 16mg vitamin C.

Chinese water chestnut has been the tuber of the sedge Eleocharis turberosa, imported in cans from Hong Kong.

Chewing gum. Gum chewing.

Chicken. Domestic fowl. Rock Cornish game hen 5–7 weeks old, 2lb; poussin, up to 6 week old, $1-\frac{1}{4}$ lb; double poussin, 8–10 weeks $1\frac{3}{4}$ –2lb; spring chicken (fryer) 12 weeks, $2-3\frac{1}{2}$–lb; roasting chicken, up to 8 months, $3\frac{1}{2}$–5lb; capon, castrated cockerel, up to 8 months, 6–8lb; boiling fowl, order animal usually after laying eggs; stag tough, boiling fowl, order animal usually after laying eggs; stag tough, male chicken up to 10 months. In recent years faster-growing strains are used to produce broilers, usually 10–12 weeks old and up to 3lb in weight.

Analysis of raw meat per 100g: 75g water, 20g protein, 4g fat, 120kcal (0.5), 0.7 mg Fe, 1mg vitamin B_6, trace vitamin B_{12} 10g free folate 2 g biotin.

Chicle. Basis of chewing gums. It is the partially evaporated of the evergreen sapodilla tree (Achra Sapota). Contains gutta (with elastic properties, consists of polumers of isoprene) and resin (triterpenes and sterols), together with carbohydrated, waxes and tannins. The same tree produces the sapodialla plum.

Chicory. Cichirium intybus. The leaves are eastern as a salad and the root, dried and partly caramelised, is often added to coffee as a diluent to cheapen the product.

The leaves are grown in the dark to disallow the development of the bitter flavour, and so are very pale in colour.

Also called succory and (in Belgium) witloof. The French call chicory ' endive belge' and endive is termed as 'chicoree' : in the USA chicory is termed as endive.

Analysis per 100g (leaf and stem) : water 96g, protein 0.8g, fat trace, carbohydrate 1.5 g (some of which is insulin), Fe 0.7 mg.

Chile Saltpetre. The common name for sodium nitrate ($NaNO_3$) used as a meat preservative.

Chili sause. Reference to a sauce which is made from

tomatoes, with spices, onions, garlic, sugar, vinegar and salt—similar to tomato catsup but containing more cayenne, onions and garlic.

Chilli. Pepper.

Chilling. The process by which food is preserved by being cooled to refrigeration temperatures, *i.e.* 0-5°C.

Chillproofing. Term used in reference to beer; treatment to prevent the appearance of haze when the beer gets chilled. Chillproofs include tannic acid to precipitate the proteins, materials like bentonite to adsorb them, and proteolytic enzymes to hydrolyse them.

Chimache. Basic Korean dish (in addition to fish and rice), having fermented cabbage with garlic, red peppers and pimientos. Vitamin C content-126mg per 100mg-led to the suggestion that the Koreans are having the highest intake of vitamin C.

Chinese Eggs. Known as pidan, houeidan and dsaoudan, according to variations in the method of preparation. Obtained by covering fresh duck eggs with a mixture of caustic soda, burnt straw ash, salt and slaked line, and storing for several months. The white and yolk coagulate and get discoloured, with practical decomposition of the protein and phospholipids.

Chinese restaurant Disease Syndrome. Refers to headache, sweating, nausea, weakness, thirst, flushing of face, abdominal pain, lachrymation—occurs occasionally when Chinese food rich in monosodium glutamate is eaten. Mild symptoms can cause from 25mg/kg weight taken on an empty stomach; results follow 25-35 min after ingestion and pass off after a few hours.

Chitin. Organic base of the hard parts of insects and crustacea, and occur also in small amounts in mushrooms. Similar in composition to cellulose but contains glucosamine instead of glucose; insoluble and indigestible.

Chitterlings. Refers to the intestine of ox, calf, or pig.

Chive. Allium schoenoprasum. A plant which is grown for its bulbs and its long thin leaves, both with a mile onion flavour, used in salads, soups and omelettes.

Chlorella. See Algae.

Chlorination. The process by which a material is treated with chlorine (CI_2).

Chlorine. As chloride ions, a mineral found with sodium in table salt and in meats, which is required for acid-base balance and for osmoregulation. The average human adult required about 5.2 grams per day and the total body content is bout 95 grams.

Free chlorine finds use as a sterilising agent—*e.g.* in drinking water.

Chlorine Dioxide. A bread 'improver'.

Chlorocrnorin. Refers to the copper-containing protein that carries oxygen in the bloodstream of the annelid worms—analogous to hemoglobin in mammals.

Chlorophyll. Refers to green colouring matter of all plant materials by the aid of which plants manufacture foodstuffs from simple salts and carbon dioxide with energy derived from sunlight, *i.e.* photosynthesis. Chlorophyll is a mixture of chlorophyll alpha and beta and two other pigments, xanthophyll and carotene.

Chlorophyllase. An enzymes which is present in all green plants, which hydrolysis chlorophyll to phytol and chlorophyllide. Reversible in action and can catalyse the synthesis of chlorophyll.

Chlorophyllide. The green colour occurring in the water offer cooking certain vegetables. The fat-soluble chlorophyll gets converted to water-soluble chlorophyllide by removal of the phytyl side-chain by alkali or enzyme.

Chocolate. A substance made from husked fermented and roasted cocoa beans which are then refined and mixed with sugar, cocoa butter flavouring, cecithin and, for milk chocolate, milk solids.

Chocolate, Drinking. Refers to partly solubilised cocoa for preparation of the beverage, including about 75% sucrose.

Analysis per 100g: 74g starch 1g N, 6g fat, 30mf Ca,

2mg Fe, 370 kcal (1.5MJ).

Cholagogue. Refers to a substance that promotes the flow of bile form the gall bladder into the duodunum.

Cholecalciferol. Vitamin D.

Cholecystokinin. A hormone which is secreted by the mucosa of the duodenum and jejunum and carried in the blood to the gall-bladder, which is thus stimulated to contract and secrete bile.

Cholelithiasis. Gallstones.

Choleretics. Refers to the substance that stimulate the secretion of bile-*e.g.* bile salts themselves taken by mouth, or cholic acid by intravenous injection.

Choline. Essential dietary factor, trimethyl hydroxyethylammonium hydroxide. It is usually classed as a vitamin, although the quantities involved are far from catalytic. Functions as a source of methyl groups and in fat transport; deficiency causes fatty infiltration of the liver; is part of the structure of the phospholipids of animal and plant tissues, Specific dietary deficiency does not occur; daily requirements not established but the daily intake is 0.5-0.5g.

Cholinesterase. Refers to the enzyme that hydrolyses acetylcholine (which is liberated by the nerve ending to stimulate muscle), so that the muscle can recover and become prepared for the next stimulus.

A number of substances, anticholinesterases, which inhibit the enzyme paralyse muscle. Examples have been war gases of the nerve group, certain insecticides and eserine, which finds use clinically in cases of excess cholinesterase (the disease myasthenia gravis).

Cholla. Loaf of white bread which is made in twist form (or Biblical beehive coil) from one large and one small piece of dough plaited together.

The dough is prepared from white flour, enriched with eggs, and a pinch of saffron, and the loaf is decorated with maw or poppy seed.

Chondroitin. Refers to a polysaccharide having galactosamine and glucuronic acid. The sulphuric acid ester, chondroitin sulphate, is found in cartilage and the organic matrix of bone. Classed as a mucopolysaccharide.

Chorleywood Bread Process. Method of obtaining dough for bread making in which the dough is submitted for increasing mechanical working (5 watt-hours or 0.4h.p. min per pound) so that, together with the help of oxidising agents, the need for bulk fermentation of the dough is eliminated. This is a 'notine' dough process and saves *i* lover 2 – hours.

Chou Pastry. Light, airy pastry which was invented by the French chef Careme, used in eclairs and profiteroles. The butter is precooked in a saucepan, then baked, Chou is French for cabbage the characteristic shaper of the cream-filled puffs.

Chowder. American term for a seafood soup; often obtained with clams or shrimps.

Chromatography. The methods used to separate different kinds of molecules and macromolecules from the one another. Most forms of chromatography rely on being able to attract solutes which are the molecules to be separated, from a solvent using a specially prepared solid material, *e.g.* paper in chromatography or silica in TLC or HPLC.

Chromium. A dietary essential in animals. Later, reduced glucose tolerance was shown in poorly nourished children which responded to chromium-containing extract of yeast, termed glucose tolerance factor (GTF), GTF is a nicotinic acid derivative of chromium and its only known function is to stimulate the enzymes involved in glucose metabolism and to facilitate the interaction of insulin with cell surface receptors.

Chromoproteins. Refers to proteins which are conjugated with a metal-containing prosthetic group-*e.g.* vertebrate hemoglobins contain iron; invertebrate hemocyains contain copper; chlorophyll contains magnesium.

Churn. To stir violently.

Chyle. Lymph rich in fat.

Chlomicrons. Droplets of unhydrolysed fat in the lymph

or blood-stream.

Chylomicrons. Droplets of unhydrolyesd fat in the lymph or blood-stream.

Chymase. Alternative name for rennin.

Chyme. Refers to partly digested mass of food as it exists in the stomach.

Chymosin. Preferred name for rennin.

Chymotrypsin. Proteolytic enzyme of the pancreatic juice; attacks parts to the protein molecule different from those attacked by pepsin and by trypsin. Secreted as the inactive precursor, chymotrypsiogen, activated by trypsin.

Cibophobia. Means dislike of food.

Cider, Cyder. An alcoholic beverage which is obtained by fermenting apple juice; contains 5-6% alcohol (by volume) and 0.7-20% sugar.

Ciguatera. Refers to poisoning from eating fish feeding in the region of coral reefs in the Caribean Sea and the Indian and Pacific Oceans. The species of fish are normally edible, and appear to derive the toxins, ciguatoxins, from their diet. Reported in seafarer's tales in the sixteenth century.

Cinnamon. Refers to the bark of various species of the genus Cinnamomum; it is split off the shoots, cured and dried. During drying the bark shrinks and curls into a cylinder or 'quill'.

Cissa. Unnatural desire for foods; alternative words, cittosis, allotriophagy and pica.

Cis-trans Isomerism. Compounds having the same molecular and structural formulae but which can exist in to geometric forms exhibit *cis-tans* isomerism. When the chemical groups in the molecule are paired on the same side, the form is *cis; on* opposite sides, it is *trans.* They are having different chemical and physical properties.

Citral. Important constituent of many essential oils, especially lemon. It is found in beta and alpha forms (*cis-and transisomers*); $C_{10}H_{16}O$. It finds use as the starting material for the synthesis of ionone (the synthetic perfume with the odour of violets), a stage in the synthesis of retinol.

Citric Acid. Tricarboxylic acid which is widely distributed in plant and animal tissue. Used as flavouring and acidulant in beverages and confectionery; provides 2.47 kcal per g. It is produced on an industrial scale by fermentation of sugars with the mould Aspergillus niger and extracted form circus fruits lemon juice contains 5-8% citric acid.

Citric Acid Cycle. Refers to the oxidation stage in the metabolism of foodstuff. Carbohydrates and fats are broken down to acetate (Active acetate or acetyl coenzyme A), and the first step in the cycle is the combination os the acety1 with oxaloacetate to form citrate. This passes through a series of reactions in which energy is released and carbon dioxide and water produced; the end-product is oxaloacetate.

As many of the amino acids can be converted into substances that lie on this pathway, the citric acid cycle has been common metabolic pathway for all three major foodstuffs. Also known as Krebs' cycle.

Citrin. Refers to mixture of two flavanones found in citrus pith, namely hesperidin and eridictin (demethylated hesperidin).

Citron. First of the citus fruits to become known to Europeans; Citrus medica. Very sensitive to cold and can be grown only in warm regions. Very thick peel; solid, sweet and acid-free pulp with practically no juice. Use for preparing candied peel.

Citronin. Flavanone glycoside which is obtained from the peel of immature Ponderosa lemons-methyoxy dihydroxy rhamno-glucoside.

Citrovorum Factor. Name given to a growth factor for the organism Leuconostoc citrovorum. It is now known to be tetrahydro-formly-pteroyl glutamic acid, which is believed to be the active form of the vitamin folic acid.

Citroxanthin. Also known as mutachrome. Yellow

carotenoid pigment in orange peel; it is having vitamin A activity.

Citrulline. An amino acid which is formed as an intermediate in the metabolism of urea in the body. Not of nutritional importance, because it is not found in food proteins.

Citrus. Genus including C. limonum (lemon), C. aurantifolia (lime), C. aurantium (sour orange), C. sinensis (sweet orange), C. medica (citron), C. nobolis (tangerine), C maxima (frapefruit), C. bergamia (begramot) and C. grandis (pomelo).

Clarification. A process which removes very small particles in colloidal dispersion from liquids. Clarification makes liquids clear and bright. The particles can be removed by filtration or the use of a chemical to form large enough particles to settle out of the liquid. *e.g.*, insinglass.

Clarifixation. Refers to the method of homogenising milk in which the cream gets separated, homogenised and re-mixed with the milk in one machine-the clarifixator.

Clarke Degrees. Water hardness.

Climacteric. The time marking the beginning of the ripening of fruit when respiration increased. Ethene which is produced by ripending fruits, controls the climacteric.

Clostridium. Genus of bacteria of which C. botulinum has been responsible for rare and often fatal form of food poisoning.

Cloudberry. Rumus chamaemorus. Golden-fruited berry growing in northern latitudes; used in similar fashion to blackberries. It is extremely rich in natural benzoic acid and the soft fruit will keep for long periods.

Clove. Refers to the dried flower buds of Caryophyllus aromaticus; mother of clove is the ripened fruit, inferior in flavour. It is having 10% fixed oil and a volatile oil, mostly eugenol, with small amounts of caryophyllene, vanillin and other substances. Used as flavour in meat products and bakery goods.

CMC. Carboxymethylcellulose.

Co I, Co II. Abbreviations of coenzymes I and II which was officially named nicotinamide adenine dinucleotide and cicotinamide adnine dinucleotide phosphate, respectively.

CoA. Abbreviation for coenzyme A.

Coacervation. Heat-reversible aggregation of amylopectin which is one explanation of the staling of bread.

Coagulase. Name given to an enzyme which is said to be present in milk and to account for the ability of milk to clot a solution of fibriogen.

Coagulation. Refers to a process whereby proteins become insoluble; effected by heat, strong acids and alkalies, metals and various other chemicals.

Coagulation takes place when, for example, an egg is cooked or a flour dough is baked.

Cobalamin. Vitamin B_{12}.

Cobalt. A mineral found in most foods, but especially meat and yeast products, which is an essential constituent of vitamin B_{12}. The average human adult require about 0.3 milligrams per day and the total body content is as little as 0.001 grams.

Cobamide. Derived from vitamin B_{12} (cobakamin) by removal of the cyano and dimethybenzimidole groups.

Coca Leaves. From the S. American plant, Erthromylon coca; having cocaine, and chewed by the natives of Peru as a stimulant.

Cocarboxylase. Refers to coenzyme that assists the enzyme carboxylase to remove carbon dioxide from various compounds, *i.e.*, decarboxylation.

Cocarboxylase has been the diphosphate of vitamin B_1 alternatively known as thiamin pyrophosphate or diphospho-Thiamin. In deficiency of vitamin B_1 the body has been unable to oxidise pyruvic acid, an intermediate stage in carbohydrate metabolism, which therefore accumulated in the blood.

Cochinequal. Red colour which is obtained from the female conchilla, Coccus cacti, found in Mexico, Central America and the West Indies. 70000 insects produce 1 lb of colour.

Legally permitted in food in most countries. It is slightly soluble in water and alcohol but hot ether.

Cock-a-leekie. Scottish soup which is made from leeks and chicken.

Cocoa Bean. The seed of the cocoa plant. They grow in pods and from the raw material from which chocolate is made. The beans are removed from the pods after fermentation which develops the flavour and colour, and chocolate, a plant fat is extracted.

Cocoa, Dutch. Cocoa which is treated with dilute solution of alkali (carbonate or bicarbonate) to improve colour, flavour and solubility. The process is known as 'Dutching'.

Cocoa Nibs. Seeds of the fruit of the cocoa plant, Theobroma cacao, are left to fement, which modifies the bitterness and the colour darkness. They are then roasted and separated from the husks as two halves of the seed known as cocoa nibs. Having about 50% fat, part of which is removed to prepare chocolate and cocoa for beverages.

Cocolait. Refers to a form of coconut 'milk' which is made by pressing coconut under high pressure and homogenising the oil and water emulsion plus coconut water (coconut milk) obtained. Bottled and used (*e.g.*, in Philippines) in place of cow's milk.

Coconut. A tropical plan, Cocos nucifera. The dried nut is copra, which is having 60-65% coconut oil. The residue after oil extraction is used for animal feed.

The hollow unripe nut is having a watery liquid known as coconut milk-which is gradually absorbed as the nut ripens.

Composition of milk from the ripe nut: 1.4% solids, 0.2% protein, 3% carbohydrate (largely sucrose).

Analysis of mature kernel per 100g: 48-80g solids, 4g protein, 35g fat, 11g carbohydrate, 4g fibre, 375 kcal (1.557MJ), 2mg Fe, traces of vitamin B_1, vitamin B_2 and nicotinic acid.

Coddle. To cook slowly in water kept just below the boiling point.

Codfish. Refers to the composition of all non-fatty fish, such as cod, hake, haddock, flatfish, is similar.

Cod fillet, per 100g; protein 16.4, fat 0.5g, kcal 75 (0.31MJ), Ca 25mg, Fe 0.7mg. vitamin A nil, vitamin B_1 0.05mg, vitamin B_2 0.08mg, nicotine acid 2.2mg, vitamin C nil.

Cod, round, per 100g: protein 7.4g, fat 0.2g, 33kcal (0.13 MJ), Ca 11mg, Fe 0.3mg, vitamin A nil, vitamin B_1 0.02mg, vitamin B_2 0.04mg, nicotinic acid 1.0 mg, vitamin C nil.

Cod Liver Oil. Oil from codfish liver; classical source of vitamins A and D, used for its medicinal properties long before the vitamins were discovered.

Average sample is having 120-1200 g vitamin A and 1-4 g vitamin D per gram.

Coeliac Disease. (Idiopathic steatorrhea, non-tropical sprue or gluteninduced enteropathy). Inherited sensitivity to the gliadin fraction of wheat (and rye and barley) flour, in which the villi of the small intensive have been severely affected and absorption of food is poor. Stools are bulky and fermenting from unabsorbed carbohydrate, and under nutrition and retarded growth result. Treatment is total exclusion of wheat, rye and barley proteins (the starches are tolerated), but rice and maize are thought to be harmless.

Coenzyme I (and II). Nicotinamide adenine dinucleotide; nicotinamide adenine dinucleotide phosphate.

Coenzyme A. Coenzyme which is used for the transfer of acetyl groups; contains the vitamin patothenic acid. Functions by its ability to combine with acetyl, forming acetyl CoA, and to transfer this to another compound. It is important in the oxidation of glucose at the stage between pyruvic acid and the citric acid cycle. And in fat metabolism.

Coenzyme Q. Ubiquinones.

Coenzyme R. Obsolete name for biotin.

Coenzymes. Refer to the substance which is needed to assist certain enzymes. They are part of the enzyme system and differ from activators in that they play no part in the activation of the substrate. Coenzymes react first with one enzyme, then with another, during the course of catalysis and so differ from prosthetic groups, which are bound to the one enzyme during the course of the reaction.

Those enzymes that do need a coenzyme have an absolute specificity for that particular coenzyme, but the same coenzyme can partner a range of enzymes. Most coenzymes are having one of the B vitamins as part of the molecule; thus Coenzyme I contains cicotinic acid. Coenzyme A contains pantothenic acid, cocarboxylase is vitamin B_1 pyrophosphate.

Co-factor. A compound needed by many enzymes to carry out the reactions which they catalyse. Many vitamins are co-factors to enzymes.

Coffee. A beverage which is produced from roasted beans from the berries of two principal types of shrub, Coffee arabica (arabica coffee) and Coffea canephora (robusta coffee). Niacin gets formed during the roasting process, and the coffee can have 10-40mg niacin per 100g, depending on the extent of roasting. Also contains caffeine, which see.

Coffee, Decaffeinated. The drug caffeine can be removed from the coffee by treating the aqueous extract of the coffee with boiling ethylene dichloride or methylene dichloride, and then drying.

Coffee Essence. Refers to aqueous extract of roasted coffee; usually about 4lb coffee per gallon of water (400*g*/*l*).

Cognac. A brandy produced in a limited area of S. France from special varieties of grape grown on shallow soil and claimed to be distilled only in pot, not continuous, stills.

Cola Drinks. Carbonated drinks having extract of cola bean, the seed of the cola tree. The seed is having caffeine. The drinks contain 3–4.5mg caffeine per fluid ounce.

Colchicine. An alkaloid which is isolated from the meadow saffron, or Autuman crocus (Colchicum). Old remedy for gout. It inhibits cell division, and used in experimental horticulture to produce plants with abnormal numbers of gens.

Cold Chain. The chain of events which affect a frozen or chilled food during its after production and before consumption. These events might include storage after production, refrigerated transport, storage before purchase, storage before use. The cold chain is extremely important in controlling the quality of a frozen or chilled food. Temperature fluctuation (change 0 during the cold chain can lead to loss of quality in frozen or chilled foods due to thawing and re-freezing, increased oxidation or growth of micro-organisms.

Cold Preservation. Campden process.

Cold Sterilisation. Irradiation; sterilisation, cold.

'Cold Store' Bacteria. Psychrophilic bacteria.

Caliform Bacteria. Refers to a group of aerobic, lactose-fermenters,.or which Escherichia coli is the most important member.

Many coliforms are not harmful, but as they arise from faeces, they are useful as a test of faecal contamination, particularly as test for water pollution.

Callagen. Refers to the soluble protein in bone, tendons, skin and connective tissue of animals and fish, converted to soluble gelatin by moist heat.

Collagen Sugar. Glycine.

Colloid. The particles (the disperse phase) suspended in a second medium (the dispersion medium). It can be solid, liquid or gas suspended in solid, liquid or gas.

Examples of gas-in-liquid colloidal systems are beaten egg white, whipped cream; of liquid-liquid colloids are emulsions such as milk, salad cream.

Colloids, lyophillic (emulsions). Refers to colloids in which there occurs a high affinity between the particles of the disperse phase and the dispersion medium. They include proteins and higher carbohydrates; very viscous; electrically charged; require large among of electrolytes for precipitation, which is reversible.

Colloids, Lyophobic. Refers to colloids in which there occurs no affinity between the particle of the disperse phase and the dispersion medium. The particles carry an electric charge and are flocculated irreversibly by electolytes. Also called suspensoids. For example, colloids of metals and inorganic salts.

Colon. Refers to last part of the intestine; consists of three parts—the ascending, the transverse and the descending colon—and finishes at the rectum.

Colony Count. A measure of microbial activity by growing a sample from contaminated food on a medium such as agar and counting the number of colonies of microorganisms after a period of growth.

Colorimeter. An instrument which is used to measure depth of colour.

Colostrum. Refers to the milk which is produced by mammals during the first few days after parturition; human colostrum contains more protein (2% compared with 1%), slightly less lactose, considerably less fat (3% compared with 5%) and overall slightly less energy than mature milk.

Colours. Refers to those which are used in foods and fall into there groups; natural pigments, mostly extracted from plant material; inorganic pigments and lakes (metals complexed with organic colours; and synthetic coal-tar dyes. Most countries permit only a limited number of these to be added to foods.

Colza Oil. Rapeseed oil.

Comminuted Meat. The meat removed from the low quality parts of the caracass after butchery, broken by machines into very small pieces or ciscous suspensions. Comminuted meat is used in the manufacture of meat products.

Comparator Block. Method of comparing colours (often used to estimate p_H).

Complan. A trade name (Glaxo laboratories) which is used for a mixture of dried skim milk, arachis oil, casein. Maltodextrins, sugar, salts and vitamins. Protein 31%, fat 16%, carbohydrate 44%, Ca 825mg, Fe 8mg per 100g, and vitamins A, B_1, B_2, nicotinic acid, vitamins B_{12}, C, D, E, K, pantothenic acid and folic acid.

Conalbumin. Refers to one of the proteins of egg-white which is comprising 12% of the total solids. Has the property of bindsing iron in an iron-protein complex that is pink. Accounts for the pinkish colour resulting when eggs are stored in rusty containers.

Concerntrated Milk. A milk which has been concentrated by evaporation of some of the water or by drying. Some concentrated milks are sweetened.

Condiment. Seasoning added to flavour foods, like salt, mustard, ginger, curry, pepper etc. Although some of these are relatively rich in nutrients, they are generally used in such small quantities that they make a negligible contribution to the diet.

Conditioning. The process in which meat is stored a low temperature (0.4°C) for several days before cooking. Conditioning is also known as aging and maturing and makes the meat more tender. Enzymes in the meat breakdown the structure of stiff actomyosin formed during rigor mortis so that the meat becomes softer.

Confectioners'Glucose. Glucose syrup.

Conge Machine. Used, in the manufacture of chocolate blend, for coating to get smoothness by kneading the material.

Cogies. Refers to the water from cooking rice, which is having much of the thiamin and nicotinic acid from the rice; used as a drink.

Conidendrin. A substance which is isolated from a number of coniferous woods whose derivatives, norconidendrin and alpha and beta conidendrol, are antioxidants. Chemically similar to the phenolic substance nordihydroguaiaretic acid.

Connective Tissue. In fish connective tissue occurs between the muscle segments (myotomes) and had the protein collagen. In meat it is spread through the muscle, uniting the muscle fibres into bundles and supporting the blood vessels (a kind of soft skeleton), and consists of both collagen and elastin. A higher content of connective tissue results in tougher meat. (Collagen is also present in bones and skin.)

On cooking, the insoluble collagen gets converted into water soluble gelatin, so making the material more tender, but elastin gets unchanged on heating. Thus, tough meat gets softened to some extent by stewing but roasting or frying is having little effect.

Consomme. A clear soup which is made from or meat extract.

Contaminated. Of foods which contain harmful substances or compounds which greatly reduce the quality of the food.

Contamination. A process by which food is made inedible, *e.g.*, by the growth of food-poisoning bacteria, moulds or yeasts, from lack of cleanliness or already contaminated food.

Controlled Atmosphere Packaging. The packaging of foods in special contaminers in which the atmosphere has been modified and can be controlled. Contain-rs used for CAP are often made of special plastics like polythene and polyamide.

Controlled Atmosphere Storage. The storage of foods, particularly fruit and vegetable, in atmospheres of controlled gas and water vapour content. The use of the correct humidity and different gases such as CO_2 can lead to the extension of the shelf-life of certain foods. CAS can be used either in large storage rooms specially designed for keeping foods or in packages which prevent the leakage of the modified atmosphere.

Convalescent Carriers. A person who excretes a food poisoning organism whilst recovering from illness caused by that organism. Excretion of the organism can continue for weeks or even years.

Convenience Food. Any food prepared by industrial processes so that it may be easily cooked and served or served cold, *e.g.*, canned foods, frozen foods, dried foods, readymade food sauces, cooki-chill foods.

Cook-freeze. The cook, chill immediately freeze foods.

Cookie. American term for biscuit.

Cooking. Required to make food more palatable and more digestible. There is breakdown of the connective tissue in meat and softening of the cellulose in plant tissues.

Broilling. Refers to cooking by direct heat over flame. US term for grilling.

Pan Broiling. Refers to cooking through hot dry metal over direct heat.

Sauteing. Cooking with small amount of fat.

Simmering. Refers to cooking in water slightly below boiling point.

Stewing. Prolonged simmering.

Fricassee. Combination of sauteing and stewing.

Devilled. Grilled or fried after coating with condiments or breadcrumbs.

Steaming. Refers to cooking by beat conveyed by steam either directly or through steam jacket, as in double boiler. Steaming also carried out above 100°C by means of pressure cookers.

Cooking, Loss of Nutrients. In general, water-soluble vitamins and minerals get lost in the cooking water, the amount depending on the surface area-volume ratio-*i.e.* greater losses take place from finely minced foods.

Fat-soluble vitamins get little affected except at frying temperatures. Proteins suffer reduction of available lysine if heated in the presence of reducing substances, and further losses under extreme conditions of temperature.

Dry heat, as in baking, causes some loss of thaiamin and of available lysine. The most sensitive nutrient by far is vitamin C, with thiamin next.

Average losses from cereals considered in standard food table to be: Boiling-40 thiamin, riboflavin, nicotinic acid, vitamin B_6 biotin and pantothenic acid; 50% total folate. Baking-5% nicotinic acid; 15% riboflavin; 25% thiamin, vitamin B_6 and pantothenic acid; 50% folate; with biotin being stable. In meat losses are approximately 20% of all the vitamins through roasting, frying and grilling and 20-60% on stewing and boiling.

Copper. A mineral found in most foods, but especially in liver, peas and beans, which is required for the formation of certain enzymes. The average human adult requires about 3.5 milligrams per day and the total body content is about 0.07 grams.

Copra. Dried coconut meat. It is used for production of coconut oil for margarine and soap.

Coprophagy. Eating of faeces. As B vitamins get synthesised by intestinal bacteria, animals that eat their faeces can make use of these vitamins.

Coriander. Refers to the dried ripe fruit of Coriandrum sativum (parsely family). Contains 20% fixed oil and 1% essential oil-largely linool or coriandrol (an isomer of geraniol). Used a flavourin meat products, bakery goods, tobacco, gin and in curry powder.

Cori Cycle. Refers to the sequence of reactions through which the liver converts lactic acid back to glycogen, namely liver glycogen-blood glucose-blood lactate-liver glycogen.

Corm. The term used for the thickened, underground base of stem of plants, often called bulbs, as, for example, taro and onion.

Corm. A generic term for cereals. It also means maize.

Corned Beef. The salt beef, *i.e.,* pickled whole meat. In many countries it is the canned product manufactured from low quality meat after partial extraction of water-soluble materials.

Analysis of canned product per 10g: 59g water, 27g protein, 12g fat 220 kcal (900kJ),1g Na, 3mg Fe, 2.5mg niacin (only trace of thiamin).

Cornflakes. Breakfast cereal which is made from maize. Apart from enriched proprietary preparations, analysis per 100g: 3g water, 7g sugars, 74g starch and dextrins, 3g dietary fibre, 8g protein, 0.5 fat, 370 kcal (1.5 MJ).

Cornflour. Purified starch from maize; in the USA called corn starch. It finds use in custard, blancmange and baking powders.

Analysis: protein 0.5%, fat 0.3%, carbohydrate 87%, fibre 0.2%, no vitamins present.

Corn Starch. See Cornflour.

Corn Steep Liquor. Refers to the first stage in the preparation of starch from maize is to soak the maize in water containing sulphur dioxide for 24th. The liquor is called corn steep liquor. It was found to be an excellent medium for growing mould to produce penicillin; the yield was greatly enhanced beyond that obtained a 'biochemical precursor' of penicillin.

Corn Sugar. Glucose.

Corn Syrup. Glucose syrup.

Corrinoids (corrins). Name assigned to chemical structure which is based on four pyrrole nuclei joined in a macro ring with three bridge carbon atoms and six conjugated double bonds. It is the basic structure of the cobalamins without the cobalt and side-chains.

Cossetters. Thin chips of sugar beet into which it gets shredded for hot-water extraction of the sugar.

Cottonseed. Of double use in the food field; the oil has been valuable as a cooking oil, for margarine when hardened, and the protein is a valuable animal feeding stuff.

Cow manure Factor. Vitamin B_{12}.

Cozymase. Nicotinamide adenine dinucleotide.

C3 Plants. Refers to the type of plants in which, during photosynthesis, the carbon dioxide is combined with ribulose diphosphate to produce two 3-carbon acids.

C4 Plants. Refers to the type of plants in which, during photosynthesis, the carbon compound, compared with 3-carbon compound in C3-type plants. The procedure concentrated the carbon dioxide and the creation is faster and more efficient than C3 photosynthesis.

Carbs. Shellfish of the suborder Brachyura of the Order Decaoda.

Edible crab, Cancer pagurus, found in shallow water among rocks; can group up to 12lb weight.

Analysis of edible portion per 100g: protein 20g, fat 5g carbohydrate 0, kcal 127 (0.53 MJ), Fe 1.3 mg, vitamin B_1 0.1 mg, vitamin B_2 0.15 mg, nicotinic acid 2.5 mg.

Cran. Measuring for herrings having 37-1/2 gallons or about 800 herrings.

Cranberry. Fleshy, acid fruit of Vaccinium oxycoccus which is resembling cherry; commonly used for cranberry sauce.

Composition per 100g : 3.5g carbobydrate, 15 kcal (0.06 MJ), 1 mg iron, 12 mg vitamin C.

Cream. Fatty part of milk. In some countries usually designated light cream, with 20-25% fat, and heavy cream, with about 40% fat. In other countries cream contains not less than 18% fat; double cream or thick cream, 48%; clotted cream, not less than 48%; whipping cream, not less than 35%.

Cream, Clotted. This usually is having a higher fat content that double cream, which legally is 48% fat. Double cream is floated in a shallow layer on a layer of skim milk and scalded. The clotted cream at 63% fat is then skimmed off. This is Devonshire cream and is having 29% water, 4% protein, 28% lactose, 0.67% ash. Cornish cream is similar but is prepared by scalding the double cream alone, not floated on a layer of milk.

Cream, Cornish. Cream, clotted.

Cream, Devonshire. Cream, clotted.

Creaming Quality. As applied to fats, it refers to the ability to absorb air during mixing.

Cream Line Index. The cream line or layer usually forms about 6% of the total depth of milk. The cream line index refers to the ratio between the percentage cream layer and the percentage fat in the milk. It is used as a test of the milk, and in ordinary bulk pasteurised milk is about 1.7.

Cream of Tartar. Potassium hydrogen tartrate. It is used with sodium bicarbonate as baking power because it acts more slowly than tartaric acid and provided a more prolonged evolution of carbon dioxide. This is tartrate baking power, similarly, phosphate baking power contains calcium acid phosphate or sodium hydrogen pyrophosphate. It is also used to 'invert' sugar in making boiled sweets.

Cream, Aleepy. Cream that will churn to butter in the normal time.

Cream, Synthetic. Name assign to:

(a) Emulsion of vegetable oil, milk or milk powder, egg yolk and sugar, and

(b) Emulsion of water with methyl cellulose, monoglycerides, and other synthetic materials.

Creatine. Methyl guanidine derivative of acetic acid. Essential part of the energy release system of muscle, as creatine phosphate, or phasphagen. Having an energy-rich bond which is released when energy is required for muscular contraction.

The anhydride of creatine is creatinine, in which form it is found in urine. Meat extract contains a mixture of the two derived from the creatine that was present in the fresh muscle. Creatine plus creatinine finds use as an index of quality of commercial meat extract, and as a measure of extract present in manufactured products, such as soups.

Creatinine. Anydride of creatine.

Cress. Lepidium sativum. Seed leaves eaten raw with mustard leaves (mustard and cress).

Cretinism. Underactivity of the thyroid gland (hypothyroidism) in children. It is resulting in poor growth and mental retardation. Hypothyrodisim in adults is myxoedema. Can result from a dietary denciency or iodine.

Crisphreads. Name given to a flour and water wafer, originally swedish and made from rye flour, but may be made from wheat flour. They are having a much lower water content then bread and some brands are richer in protein because of added wheat gluten.

Although it is popularly believed to be an air in slimming, they give more energy than the same weight of orcinary bread, as they contain less water.

Cristal Height. Refers to a measure of leg length taken from the floor to the summit of the iliac crest. Cristal height as a proportion of total height gets increased with age in children, and a reduced rate of increase has been an indication of undernourishment.

Cross-infection. The way in which a camer of a food poisoning organism can spread it to other individuals, *e.g.*. the spread of Salmonella infection between battery chickens.

Croutons. Refers to the small diced or shaped pieces of bread fried in fat.

Crude Fibre. The indigestible part of food left other nutrients have been digested and absorbed in the body. Crude fibre in foods can be measured after extraction (p.90) with dilute acid followed by dilute acid followed by dilute alkali. In recent years fibre has been shown to be necessary in the diet. Diets low in fibre are thought to lead to such illnesses as heart disease and atheroscelerosos as well as diseases of the alimentary canal.

Crumb. The solid structure within baked bread surrounding the trapped bubbles of carbon dioxide.

Cryogenic cooling. A process of cooling to chill or freezing temperatures using liquid nitrogen.

Cryogenic Freezing. Freezing using extremely cold freezants like boiling nitrogen or boiling or subliming carbon dioxide.

Cryptoxanthin. Yellow colouring matter in certain vegetables like yellow maize, and in the seeds of physalis, the Chinese Lantern. A hydroxy derivative of carotene. It is converted into retinol in the body.

Crystallin. Protein of the lens of the eye.

Crytallized Fruit. A traditional method of preserving fruit particularly in the Middle East Fruits are cut into pieces which are coated in concentrated solutions of sugar. This causes dehydration of the fruit pieces through osmosis of water out of the plant tissue.

CSM. Corn-soya-milk; protein-rich baby food (20% protein) made from 68% precooked maize (corn), 25% defatted soya flour and 5% skin milk powder, with added vitamins B_1, B_2, B_6, B_{12}, nicotinic acid, pantothenic acid, folio acid, vitamins A, D and E, and calcium carbonate.

Cubs. Trade name (Nabisco Foods Ltd) for a breakfast cereal made from wheat.

Cucumber. Fruit of Cucumis sativus. It is member of the gourd family.
Analysis per 100g: protein 0.6g, fat 0.1g, kcal 10 (0.04MJ), Ca 7mg, Fe 0.2mg, vitamin B_1 0.02mg, vitamin B_2 0.03mg, nicotinic acid 0.1 mg, vitamin C. 6mg.

Cucurbits. Term used for vegetable of the Cucurbitacease.

Culture. (n) A group or collection of bacteria or other micro organisms.

Cultured Milk Product. Any milk product made by the addition of harmless micro-organisms *e.g.*, yoghurt.

Cumin Seed. Dried fruit of Cuminum cyminum (parsely family). It contains about 10% fixed oil and 2-4% essential oil, largely cuminal. Used in curry powder and for flavouring cordials.

Curacao. Liqueur which is made from the rind of seville oranges and brandy or gin; 30% alcohol, 30% sugar.

Curds. Clotted protein formed when fresh milk gets treated with rennet; the fluid left is whey.

Curd Tension. Refers to measure of the toughness of the curd formed from milk by the digestive enzymes. It is used as an index of the digestibility of the milk. The sample gets coagulated with rennin and the force needed to pull a knife blade through the curd is measured in grams under standardised conditions. Ideal score has been zero, below 20 satisfactory. Cow's milk 46; diluted with equal colume of water 20; reconstituted spray-dried milk 10; reconstitued rollerdried milk 5; evaporated milk 3; human milk 1.

Curing of Meat. The term used for a method of preservation by treating with salt and sodium nitrate (and nitrite), which serves to inhibit growth of pathogenic organisms while salt-tolerant bacteria develop. During the pickling process the nitrate gets converted into nitrite, which combines with the muscle pigment, myoglobin, to form the red-coloured nitrosomyoglobin characteristic of pickled meat products.

Currants. Fruit of Ribes species; white, red and black.

Analysis per 100g: Redcurrants: protein 1.1g. carbohydrate 4.4g, water 83g kcal 21 (0.09 MJ), Fe 1.2mg, vitamin C 4mg.

White currants; protein 1.3g, carbohydrate 5.6g, water 83%, kcal 26 (0.11 MJ), Fe 1mg, vitamin C 40mg.

Curry. Refers to the mixture of several spices, including turmeric, coriander, cardamom, cumin fenugreek, ginger, mustard, chilli, cloves and peeper. Reported to contain up to 75-100mg iron per 100g but a large part of this is due to contamination.

There is also curry plant (Murraya koenigii) number of alkaloids.

Custard. May refer to custard powder, or to egg custard. Egg custard is composed of milk and egg cooked together.

Custards Apple. Refers to one of a number of species of tropical American trees of the family Anonocease. Sour sop, Anoma muricata, white fibrous flesh less, sweet than the others, fruit may weigh 6 to 8lb; sweet sop (A. squamosa) also known as 'true' custard apple, popular in West Indies ; bullock's heart (A. reticulata), buff coloured flesh.

Analysis per 100g : 22g carbohydrate, 1g protein, 93 kcal (0.45MJ), 0.5mg Fe, 0.1 mg vitamin B_1, 0.08 mg vitamin B_2, 0.8mg nicotinic acid, 30mg vitamin C.

Custard Powder. Generally maize starch, coloured and flavoured.

Cyanocobalamin. Vitamin B_{12}.

Cyclamate. Sodium cyclo-Hexyl-sulphamate. A chemical sweetner 30 times sweeter than sucrose. Cyclamate is now banned for use in foods in many countries because it is known to be a possible carcinogen.

Cyelitols. Cyclic sugar such as inositiols, quercitols and tetritols.

Cyclo-hexyl-sulphamate, Sodium. Refers to non-nutritive sweetner. It is 30 times as sweet as sugar, also used as the calcium salt; synthesised 1997.
Useful in low-calorie foods. Also called cyclamate and Sucaryl (trade name). Unlike saccharine, it is stable to heat.

Cysteine. Refers to a sulpher-containing non essential amino acidamino thiol propionic acid. Cystine gets formed when two molecules of cystene are reduced and linked via the -S-S-bond.
Cysteine is used as dough 'improver'.

Cystic Fibrosis. Refers to an inborn error of metabolism which causes a disturbance of the exocrine glands, with failure to secrete pancreatic enzymes, so that food is incompletely digested and absorbed. It can be treated by feeding predigested protein or adding dried pancreatin to the diet.

Cystine. The double molecule of reduced cystine, linked via the -S-S bond. It forms about 12% of hair protein, keratin.

Cytochrome. Refers to pigment present in every type of licing cell (except the strictly anaerobic bacteria). It acts as an intermediate hydrogen acceptor in passing hydrogen along the chain from the substrate to oxygen, the ultimate hydrogen acceptor.

Cytochrome P450. Refers to part of the detoxication system of the body; at least four enzymes are involved-cytochromes P450 and b_5 together with their reductases. About ten forms of P450 take place in the liver and the system as a whole is referred to as mixed function oxidases; can deal with a variety of substrates, including drugs and food additives.

Cytokinins. Refers to substances the stimulate cell division-cytokinesis- and control development of plants; found in seed embryos, developing fruits and buds. They are derivatives of the purine base adenine.

D

Damson. Refers to small dark-blue plum, Prunus damascena.
Analysis per 100g: protein 0.5g, water 70g, carbohydrate 8.6g, kcal 34 (0.14MJ), Fe 0.4mg, vitamin B_1 0, 1mg, nicotinic acid 0.25 mg.

Dandelion Greens. Refers to the leaves of the weed. Leontodon taraxacum, used sometimes as a salad.
Analysis per 100g; protein 2.4g fat 0.6g, Ca 135mg, Fe 2.8mg, kcal 40(0.17MJ), carotene 3000g. vitamin B_1 0.17mg, vitamin B_2 0.13 mg, nicotinic acid 0.7 mg, vitamin C 25 mg.

Dark Adaptation. Refers to the change that takes place in the retina of the eye to assist vision in dim light. In dark adaptation a pigment, visual purple or rhodopsin, is formed from retinal (vitamin A aldehyde) and a protein. This is bleached in bright light. When body stores of retinol are inadequate, poor dark adaptation-night blindness-results. This is the earliest indication of vitamin A deficiency.

Dasheen. West Indian name for taro.

Date-plum. Persimmon.

Date. Refers to fruit of date palm, Phoenix dactylifera, known as far back as 3000 B.C. Three types: 'soft' (about 80% of dry matter is invert sugars): 'semi-dry' about 40% of dry matter is invert sugars and about 40% is sucrose) : 'dry' (20-40% of dry matter is invert sugars, 40-60% sucrose).

General analysis per 100g : 15g water, 9g dietary fibre, 2g, protein, 65g sugars, 250 kcal (IMJ), 1.5 mg iron, small amounts of most of the Vitamin.

DBD Process. Dry-banch-dry process.

DE. Dextrose equivalent value.

Decimal Reduction Time. The time taken to reduce the number of micro-organisms in a food sample to one tenth of the original among when heating at a constant temperature.

Defibrinated Blood. Blood, defibrinated.

Degumming Agents. The substances which are used in refining of fats of remove mucilaginous matter consisting of gum, resin, proteins and phosphatides, include hydrochloric and phosphoric acids, and phosphates.

Dehydroacetic Acid. Also sodium salt (DHA-S). It has been found to be active against moulds but not a permitted additive.

Chemically it is the condensation product of acetic and acetoacetic acids, or 3-acetyl-6-methy;-1-pyran-2,4 dione.

Dehydroascorbic Acid. Oxidised form of vitamin C which can readily get reduced to the ordinary form, and is therefore biologically active.

Dehydrocanning. Refers to a process in which 50% of the water is removed from a food before canning. The advantages are that the texture gets retained by the partial dehydration and there is a saving in bulk and weight.

Dehydrocholesterol. Vitamin D.

Dehydrofreezing. Refers to a process which is used for preservation of fruits and vegetables by evaporation of one-half to two-thirds of the water before freezing. The texture and flavour are claimed to be superior to those resulting from either dehydration or freezing alone, and rehydration more rapid than with dehydrated products.

Dehydrogenases. Refers to the enzymes that carry out oxidations in the living cell by removing hydrogen from the substrate. They can only function by passing this hydrogen on to another substance, called the intermediate hydrogen acceptor. It is ultimately passed on to oxygen to form water.

Specific dehydrogenases are known for each substrate-e.g. succinic dehydrogenase, lactic, malic glucose, etc.

Dehydrogenation. Intermediate hydrogen carrier; oxidase; oxidation.

Dehydroretinol. Formerly termed vitamin A.

Demerare Sugar. Sugar.

Demersal Fish. Refers to those found living on or near the bottom of the sea, including cod, haddock, whiting and halibut, which contain little oil, 1-4%.

Denature. To bring about changes in protein structure, often with loss of function including the loss of native conformation. Heat violent shaking changes in pH and ultraviolet light can make proteins denature. Sometimes these changes can be reversed to give the native conformation.

Denaturation.

1. Refers to a reversible change in proteins that precedes coagulation (which the solubility is reduced and fee-SH groups appear. Denaturation can be carried out by changes in pH, heat, ultraviolet irradiation and violent agitation.)

There occurs no change in nutritive value, but pharmacological activity is often lost.

2. When the term is applied to alcohol, it implies the addition of denaturing agents, such as methyl violet and pyridine (as in methylated spirits) to render it unpleasant and so prevent its consumption.

Dentritic Salt. Refers to a form of ordinary table salt, sodium chloride, with the crystals branched or star-like (dendritic) instead of the normal cubes. The advantages claimed include the lower bulk density, rapid solution, and unusual capacity for absorbing moisture before becoming wet.

Deodorisation. Generally this term is applied to the removal of flavour (as in deodorised fish meal) but more specifically it is applied to the deodorisation of facts during refining. Superheated steam is bubbled through the hot oil under vacuum when most of the flavoured substances get distilled off.

Depectinisation. Refers to the removal of pectins from fruit pulp to produce a clear thin juice instead of a viscours, cloudy liquid: achieved by the used of enzyme preparations.

Derbyshire Neck. Goitre; iodine.

Descriptor. A word used to describe a quality in food samples during a descriptive test. Descriptors are usually agreed by the judges before a test.

Desferrioxamine. An iron-chelating agent which is used medicinally to reduce iron content of the body.

Desmosine. Refers to a complex cross-linked compound which is involving four lysyl residues formed, together with isodesmosine, in connective tissue.

Desoxyribonucleic Acid. Nucleic acids.

Deterioration. The process in which food quality is reduced due to spoilage bad treatment or poor storage.

Detoxication. The process in which food quality is reduced due to spoilage, bad treatment or poor storage.

Detoxication. Means destruction of a toxic compound, or more usually, alteration of a chemical group to produce a non-toxic product.

In the body detoxication gets effected by oxidation, reduction, hydrolysis; or by combination (conjugation) with glycine, glucuronic acid, glutamine, cysteine; or by methylation. For example, the toxic substance benzoic acid is excreted in the urine as a complex with glycine, namely hippuric acid.

Devitalised Gluten. Gluten.

Dewberry. Refers to a large variety of blackberry, but different in flavour.

Dexedrine. Anoretic drugs.

Dextran. Refers to a polysaccharide which is composed of linked fructose units; unwelcome in the Sugar factory but valuable clinically for blood transfusion (plasma extender). Produced by the action of Betacoccus arabinosus on sugar.

Dextrins. Mixture of soluble compounds which get formed by partial breakdown of starch by heat, acid or enzymes (complete breakdown yields maltose). Formed when bread gets toasted.

Nutritionally equivalent to starch; industrially used as adhesives in the sizing of paper and textiles, and as gums.

Dextrorotatory. Optical activity.

Dextrose. Alternative name for glucose. Commercially the term glucose's usually used to mean corn syrup (a mixture of glucose, sugars and dextrins) and pure glucose is called dextrose.

Dextrose Equivalent Value. This term is used to indicate the degree of hydrolysis of starch into glucose syrup. It is defined as the total reducing sugar content expressed as dextrose, calculated as a percentage of the dry solids content (i.e., the higher the DE the more sugar and the less dextrins are present).

Liquid glucoses are commercially available ranging from 2 DE to 65 DE. A complete acid hydrolysis converts all the starch into glucose but produces bitter degradation products.

Glucose syrups above 55 DE are called 'high conversion' (of starch); 35-55, regular conversion. Below 20 the products of hydrolysis are maltins or maltodextrins.

Dhals. Indian term which is used for split peas of various kinds, e.g., pigeon pea (Cajanus indicus), khesari (Lathyrus sativus), red dahl or Massur dhal is the lentil (Lens esculenta).

Diabetes, Alloxan. Alloxan.

Diabetes Mellitus (sugar diabetes). Refers to a metabolic disorder which is affecting mainly carbohydrate metabolism; as inability metabolise glucose, which therefor appears in the urine. Usually occurs due to a deficiency of insulin and be treated by insulin injection (also possibly due to increased destruction of insulin in the body, treated by oral drugs such as tolbutamide).

Impaired glucose metabolism gives rise to excessive fat breakdown, with accumulation of the penultimate products of fatty acid oxidation-namely acetoacetic acid, betahydroxbutyric acid and acetone (the so-called ketone bodies). These can cause diabetric coma.

Diabetes, Renal. Refers to the appearance of glucose in the urine without undue elevation of the blood sugar. It occurs due to reduction of the renal threshold which allows the blood glucose to be excreted.

Diabetes Text. Glucose tolerance.

Di-acetate, Sodium and Calcium. Used to inhibit the growth of moulds in foods. Permitted in some countries. Chemical formula $CH_3COON^aCH_3COOH.1/2H_2O$ (equimolecular compound of acetic acid and sodium acetate).

Diacetyl. $CH_2COCOCH_3$. Refers to the flavour-aroma agent in butter, formed during the ripening stage by the organism Streptococcus lactis cremoris. Added as a synthetic compound to margarine as 'butter flavour'.

Dialysis. Refers to the separation of small molecules from larger in solution by virtue of their different rates of diffusion through a membrane. Membranes are natural, such as pig bladder, or artificial, such as cellulose derivatives or collodin.

The solution is usually kept in a bag of the membrane and this immersed in water. The small molecules diffuse out into the water, leaving the large molecules inside the bag. It is a frequent method of separating proteins from solutions of salts.

Diaphorase. Refers to a flavoprotein enzyme in the cell respiratory system: its function is to accept hydrogen from Nadh to become Nadph.

Diastase. Amylases.

Diastatic Activity. Of flour; this term refers to a measure of its ability to produce sugar from its own starch under the influence of its own diastase. This sugar is required for the growth of the yeast during the fermentation. Measured as 'maltose figure'.

Dicoumarn. Refers to a toxic substance which is found in spoiled sweet clover causes haemorrhage (haemorrhagic sweet clover disease) by interfering with the synthesis of prothrombin in the liver, i.e., has an anti-vitamin K action. It is used clinically to prenent postoperative thrombosis.

Dietary Fibre. Fibre, dietary.

Dietatic Foods. Foods which are prepared to meet the particular nutritional needs of persons whose normal processes of assimilation or metabolism are modified, or for whom a particular effect is to be obtained by a controlled intake of foods or certain nutrients. They may be formulated for persons suffering from physiological disorders or for healthy people with additional needs.

Diethyl Pyrocarbonate. Pyrocarbonic acid diethyl (trade name Baycovin). It is used as a preservative for wines, soft drinks and fruit juices at a level of 50-300ppm. Breaks down within a few days to ethanol and carbon dioxide; does not inhibit moulds.

Dietitian, Dietician. Refers to one who applies the principles of nutrition to the feeding of individuals and groups; plans menus and special diets, supervises the preparation serving of meals; instructs in the principles of nutrition as applied to the selection of foods.

Diets. Under Hey diet; Karell diet; Kempner diet; Ketogenic diet; Lenghartz diet; meulingracht diest; Salisbury cure; salt-free diets; Sippy diet.

Diets, Therapeutic. Therapeutic diets.

Differential Cell Count. Leucocytes.

Digester. Alternative name for autoclave or pressure cooker.

Digestibility. The amount of food which is absorbed form the digestive tract into the blood stream, usually about 90-95%. Digestibility is measured as the difference between intake of food and output of waste from the body.

Digestion. Refers to the breakdown of a complex into its constituent parts. Most frequently refers to the digestion of food, which implies the breakdown by the digestive enzymes of proteins to amino acids, starch to glucose, fats to glycerol and fatty acids-these simple breakdown products are then absorbed into the bloodstream. Digestion is also applied to the acid hydrolysis of a protein; the Kjeldhal digestion is the complete breakdown of a nitrogenous compound to ammonia by sulphuric acid.

Digestive Juices. Bile; gastric secretion; intestinal juice; pancreatic juice.

Dihydrochalcones. Neohesperidin.

Dilatation of fats. When fats change from solids to liquid at the same temperature there occurs an increase in volume. Measurement of this increase, dilatometry, is used to estimate the amount of solid far present in a mixture at any given temperature. The precise measure refers to the difference between the volumes of the solid and the liquid fat measured in microlitres per 25g of fat.

Dill. Dried ripe fruit of Anthem graveolens (Parsley family); leafy tops also used. Having 15% fixed oil and 2-4% essential oil containing carvone, limonene and termpenes. Used in pickles and soups.

Diose. Disaccharides.

Dipeptide. Polypeptide.

Diphenyl. This, and orthopheylphenol (OPP), find use for treatment of fruit after harvesting to prevent mould growth. Permitted in citrus fruit, diphenyl up to 110ppm, OPP up to 70ppm. Apples, pears and pineapples may contain 10ppm, peaches 20ppm, and melons 125ppm of OPP.

Diphosphopyridine Nucleotide. Nicotinamide Adenine Dinucleotide.

Diphophothiaman. Cocarboxylase.

Dipsa. Foods that cause thirst. Dipsetic-tending to produce thirst.

Dipsesls. Also dipsosis. Extreme thirst, craving for abnormal kinds of drinks. Dipsomania-imperative morbid craving for alcoholic drink.

Dipsogen. Refers to thirst-provoking agent.

Direct Extract. Meat extract.

Disaccharide Intolerance. Refers to the impaired ability to digest maltose, sucrose or lactose, which may be inherited. Generalised lactose intolerance may be an adaptation to the absence of milk from the diet, and can be secondary to various inflammatory and degenerative diseases of the small intestine.

Treatment is by omitting the offending sugar from the diet.

Disaccharides. Sugars which are composed of two monosaccharide molecules combined, with the elimination of a molecule of water. For example, glucose, $C_6H_{12}O_6$, plus fructose, $C_6H_{12}O_6$, produces sucrose, $C_{12}H_{22}O_{11}$. Conversely, when a disaccharide gets hydrolysed, either by acid or enzymically, a molecule of water gets added and two monosaccharides result.

Also known as dioses or disaccharoses.

Disaccharose. Disaccharides.

Disc Mill. One or more revolving circular plates between which substances, e.g. foodstuffs, are ground. The discs can be separated by projecting teeths or pins, used to grind grain, fruit, sugar, chocolate, pastes, etc.

Discrimination Test. Sensory analysis in which the difference between food samples are judged, e.g. paired comparison test tangle test duo-trio test, taste threshold test.

Distiller's Solubles. Spent wash.

Diuresis. Loss of water which occurs from the body as urine.

Diuretics. Refers to the substances that increase the secretion of urine; include organic mercury compounds, xanthines (therefore also coffee and tea) and substances that alter the alkaline reserve of the blood, such as urea, potassium nitrate, potassium chloride.

Djenkolic Acid. A sulphur-containing amino acid which occurs in the djenkol bean, Pithecolobium lobtaum (grown in parts of Sumatra). It is similar to cysteine in structure; it gets metabolised but because it is relatively insoluble, and djenkolic acid that escapes metabolism can crystallise in the kidney tubes and cause damage.

DNA. Desoxyribonucleic acid.

Dockage. Name of a foreign material in wheat which can be readily removed by a simple cleaning procedure.

Do-maker Process. For continuous breadmaking. Ingredients have been automatically fed into continuous dough mixer, the yeast suspension being added in a very active state.

Dough. The characteristically dry paste made from cereal flour which is cooked to make breads and bread-like goods, e.g., rills. Yeast may be added to dough in order to act as a raising or leavening agent. The yeast ferments in the dough producing carbon dioxide which causes the dough to fill with small bubbles and so, to rise.

Dough Cakes. Term is used to include crumpets, muffins and pikelets, all made from flour, water and milk; batter is raised with yeast and baked on a hot plate. Crumpets have sodium bicarbonate added to the batter; muffins are thick and well aerated, less tough than crumpets; pikelets are made from crumpet batter that has been thinned down.

Douglas Bag. Inflatable bag which is used for collecting expired air, energy usage can be determined from the oxygen and carbon dioxide analysis, i.e., by indirect calorimetry.

Dough Development. The process in dough making in which gluten form in the wheat flour. The yeast, which is added to the dough mixture, is allowed to ferment, produces carbon dioxide gas and the dough rises.

$C_6H_{12}O_6 \rightarrow 2C_2H_5OH + 2XO_2$

DPN. Nicotinamide Adenine Dinucleotide.

Drip. The process by which liquid is lost from meat during storage after butchery. Also used as the name of the liquid lost from the meat.

Dripping. Unbleached and untreated fat from the fatty tissues or bones of sheep or oxen.

Drupes. Botanical name for fruit that is single seed which is surrounded by stony and fleshy pericarp, e.g. apricot, cherry, plum.

Dry-blanch-dry Process . Refers to a method of drying fruit so as to retain the bright colour and flavour, it is faster than drying in the sun and preserves flavour and colour better than hot air drying. The material can be dried to 50% water at about 82°C, blanched for a few minutes, then dried at 68°C over a period of 6-24h to 15-20% water content.

Dry Curing. A process of curing meat with solid salt rather than brine.

Dryers. Fluid bed dryer; pneumatic dryer; roller dryer; rotary louver dryer; spray dryer.

'Dry Frying'. Frying without using fat by using an anti-stricking agent of silicone or a vegetable extract.

Dry Ice. Solid carbon dioxide. It has a temperature of -79°C. It is used to refrigerate foodstuffs in transit, for carbonation of liquids, and for cold trapin the laboratory. Sublimes from the solid stage to a gas without liquefying; latent heat at subliming temperature 246 BTU per pound; available refrigeration per pound nearly twice that of ice.

Drying, Axeotrople. Azeotrope.

Drying Oil. Refers to highly unsaturated oil that absorbs oxygen and, when in thin films, polymerises to form a skin. Linseed and tung oil are examples of drying oils used in pains and in the manufacture of linoleum. Nutritionally these oils have been similar to edible fats, but when polymerised, are toxic.
Also iodine, value.

Du Bois Formula. Surface area.

Ductless Glands. Hormones.

Dulcin. Synthetic material, parphenetylurea (paraphenetolcarbamide). It is 250 times as sweet as sugar but not permitted in foods. Discovered 1883; also termed as sucrol and valzin.

Dulcite. Dulcitol.

Dulcitol. Refers to a six-carbon sugar-alcohol formed by reduction of galactose. Occurs in Madagascar manna (Melampyrum nemorosum), and also known as melampyrin, dulcite and galacticol.

Dulse. Purplish-red edible seaweed which is eaten raw or cooked.

Dun. In salted fish refers to the brown discoloration caused by mould growth.

Dunst. Very fine semolina (i.e. starch from the endosperm of the wheat grain) approaching the fineness of flour. Also termed as break middlings (not to be confused with middlings, which is the branny offal).

Duodenum. Refers to first part of the small intestine, between the stomach and the jejunum. Pancreatic juice and bile are secreted into the intestine and the major part of digestion takes place there.

Duo-trio Test. A test similar to the triangle test in that three samples are used. In this case the person is asked to say which of two samples is different from a control sample.

Durian. Durio zibethinus; tropical fruit with disgusting odour.

Durum Wheat. Refers to a hard type of wheat of the species Tricitum durum (most bread wheats are Tricitum vulgare). It is largely used for the production of semolina intended for the preparation of macaroni.

Dutch Oven. Semicircular metal shield which may be placed close to an open fire; fitted with shelves on which food is roasted. It may also be clamped to the fire bars.

D Value. Decimal reduction time.

Dyox. Trade name for chlorine dioxide used to treat flour.

Dyspepsia. Refers to any pain or discomfort associated with eating. Dyspepsia may be a symptom of gastritis, peptic ulcer, gallbladder disease, etc., or, if there is no structural change in the intestinal tract, it is called 'functional dyspepsia'. Treatment includes a bland diet.

E

Ecuelle. Device for getting peel oil from citrus fruit. Consists of a shallow funnel lined with spikes on which the fruit is rolled by hand. As the oil glands are pierced, the oil and cell sap collect in the bottom of the funnel.

Eddo. West Indian name for taro.

EDTA. Ethylenediamine Tetraacetic acid.

EFA. Essential fatty acids, which see.

Egg. Hens' eggs are graded according to quality and size:

Quality: A-fresh; A extra-packed less than 7 days ago; B-less fresh than A, preserved or refrigerated; C-fit for food manufacture only.

Sizes: Grade 1, 70g and over, then grades 2 to 6 at 5g intervals, with grade 7 under 45g.

Analysis whole egg per 100g: 12g protein, 11g fat, 150kcal (0.60MJ), 50mg Ca, 2mg Fe, 150mg retinol. 0.1mg vitamin B_1 0.5μg vitamin B_2, 0.1mg nicotinic acid, 2μg vitamin D 1.6mg vitamin E.

Yolk per 100g : 16g protein, 31g fat, 340 kcal (1.4MJ) 130mg Ca, 6mg Fe, 400μg retinol, 0.3mg vitamin B, 0.5mg vitamin B, 0.02mg nicotinic acid, 5μg vitamin D, 5mg vitamin E.

White per 100g : 9g protein, trace fat, 36 kcal (0.15MJ), 5mg Ca, trace Fe, 0.4mg vitamin B, 0.1mg nicotinic acid. Useful in food preparation to thicken sauces and custards, as an emulsifier, to hold air in meringues and sponges, and as binder in croquettes.

Egg Albumin. Egg-white.

Egg, Dehydrated. Analysis per 100g : 43g protein, 43g fat, 500 kcal (2MJ), 190mg Ca, 8mg Fe, 500ug retinol, 0.35mg vitamin B, 1.2mg vitamin B, 0.2mg nicotinic acid, 6μg vitamin D, 6mg vitamin E.

Egg plant. Aubergine.

Egg Proteins. Refers to a mixture of individual proteins, including ovalbumin, ovomucin, ovoglobulin, conalbumin and vitellin. Egg-white contain 10.9% protein, mostly ovalbumin; yolk contains 16% protein, mainly two phosphoproteins-vitellin and vitellenin.

Egg Substitute. Name formerly used for golden raising powder.

Egg-white. 87.8% water, 10.8% protein, 0.6% ash. Composed of outer layer of thin white, layer of thick white, richer in ovomucin, and inner layer of thin white surrounding the yolk. Eggs vary in ratio of thick to thin white, depending on the individual hen. Higher percentage of thick white desirable for frying and poaching (helps the egg to coagulate into small firm mass instead of spreading); thin white produces larger volume of froth when beaten than does thick.

Proteins are ovomucin, ovalbumin, ovomucoid, ovoglobulin and conalbumin.

EH. Equilibrium humidity.

Einkorn. Refers to a type of wheat, the wild form of which, Triticum boeoticum, was probably one of the ancestors of all cultivated wheats. Still grown in some parts of S. Europe and Middle East, usually for animal feed.

The name einkorn, 'one seed', derives from the single seed found in each spikelet.

Eiweiss Milch. Protein milk.

Elastin. Insoluble protein which is uniting muscle fibres in meat, not changed in heating; the causes of tough meat.

Elastin. Insoluble protein which is uniting muscle fibres in meat, not changed in heating; the cause of tough meat.

Electron Microscope. An instrument which can magnify

objects up to over a million times their actual size using a beam of electrons.

Electrophoresis. Refers to the movement of electrically charged particles under the influence of a current. The electric charge on proteins is sufficient to make them migrate at a rate depending on the protein itself, and electrophoreses on paper, gels, etc., is a convenient analytical tool for separating proteins.

Electropure Process. Refers to a method of pasteurising milk by passing a low-frequency, alternating current.

Elemental Diet. Defined diet formula which is prepared from purified substances (amino acids, peptides, glucose) which requires little digestion and leaves minimum residue; used in oral or tube feeding.

Embden-meyerhof-parnas Scheme. Name for the first series of steps in the breakdown of glucose in the tissues, as far as pyruvic acid, i.e., the glycolytic part as distinct from the subsequent oxidation.

Emblic. Berry of the S.E. Asian malacca tree, Emblica officinalis; similar in appearance to the gooseberry. Also known as Indian gooseberry. Rich source of vitamin C-600mg per 100g.

Emmer. Refers to a type of wheat known to be used more than 8000 years ago; tetraploid (4 sets of 7 chromosomes). Wild emmer is Triticum dicoccoides and true emmer is T. dicoccum. Nowadays usually grown for animal feed.

Emulsifier. A substance which allows the mixing of two or more immiscible liquids to form a stable emulsion. Emulsifiers work by coating the surface of droplets of one liquid in such a way that they can stay dispersed in the second liquid.

Emulsifying Agents. Substances like gums, egg yolk, albumin, casein, soaps, agar, lecithin, glycerol monostearate, alginates, Irish moss, which are used to aid the uniform dispersion of oil in water, i.e., form emulsions like margarine, ice-cream, salad cream, etc. Stabilisers maintain these emulsions in a stable form. Also used in baking to aid the smooth incorporation of fat into the dough and to keep the crumb soft.

Emulsifying Salts. Sodium, citrate, sodium phosphates and sodium tartrate which are used in the manufacture of milk powder, evaporated milk, sterilised cream and processed cheese.

Emulsion. Mixture of glycosidase enzymes in bitter almond which decompose the glucoside amygdalin to benzaldehyde, glucose and hydrocyanic acid.

Emulsion. Refers to an intimate mixture of two immiscible liquids, one being dispersed in the other in the form of the droplets. For example, oil and water. They will stay mixed only as long as they are stirred together unless an emulsifying agent (which see) is added to stabilise the emulsion.

Endergonic. Used of reactions (in living tissues) that need a supply of energy, such as the synthesis of complex molecules.

Endive. Refers to a species of chicory, Cichorium endiva; the curly leaves are eaten as a salad. Called chicory in the USA.

Analysis per 100g : water 94g, protein 1.8g carotene 2000µg, vitamin C 12mg.

Endomorph. A short, well-built person. Not a very widely used word in modern nutrition.

Endopeptidases. Enzymes that are able to split peptide bonds inside the protein molecule; i.e., according to the older nomenclature, they are proteinases, such as pepsin, trypsin and chymotrypsin.

Endosperm. Refers to the inner and greater part of cereal grains. In wheat comprises about 83% of the grain, mainly starch, and is the sources of semolina (which see). Contains only about 10% of the thiamin, 35% of the riboflavin, 40% of the nicotinic acid, 50% of the pyridoxine and pantothenic acid of the whole grain.

Endotoxins. Refers to toxins which are produced by bacteria as integral part of the cell, so cannot be separated; unlike endo toxins, they do not usually stimulate antitoxin formation but the antibodies produced act directly on the bacteria. Unlike exotoxins, they are relatively stable to heat.

Energy. Defined as the ability to do work. Exists in several forms, such as chemical energy in fuels and food; kinetic, potential, light and heat energy. Measured in joules. As various forms of energy are interconvertible, generally measured as heat in calories or British thermal units. Total chemical energy in a food, as released in the bomb calorimeter, is gross energy. After allowance is made for the losses in the faeces the remainder is digestible energy. After allowance is made for loss in the urine (e.g., urea from dietary proteins) the remainder is metabolisable energy. Finally, after allowing for the loss by specific dynamic action, the remainder is net energy. Available energy in foods can be calculated by use of the following factors: protein 17kj/g, fat 37 kj/g, carbohydrate (calculated as monosaccharide) 16kj/g, alcohol 29kj/g. Energy expenditure of average adult man: basal 1700kcal (701 MJ) per day; light work, total 2300 kcal (9.7 MJ); medium work 3000 kcal (12.6 MJ) ; heavy work 3500 kcal (14.7 MJ).

Energy Conversion Factors. Refers to the amount of energy available in foodstuffs. When this was expressed in calories, the factors were slightly different, depending upon whether allowances were made for absorption. With the change to the joule it was recognised that conversion factors for calculating the metabolisable energies of foods are relatively inaccurate, and until better values become available the following are used; protein 17kh/g, fat 37kj/g, carbohydrate (ad monosaccharide) 16kj/g, ethyl alcohol 29kj/g.

Enfleurage. The term used for the method of extracting essential oils from blossoms, by placing them on glass trays covered with purified lard or other fat, which eventually becomes saturated with the oil.

Enocianina. Desugard grape extract which is used to colour fruit flavours. It is prepared by acid extraction of skins of red grapes; bluish when neutralised, turns red on acidifying.

Enolase. Refers to an enzyme that catalyses the conversion of 2 phosphoglyceric acid to phospho-enol-pyruvic acid, with the formation of an energy-rich phosphate bond. Important in the breakdown of glucose.

Enrichment. Term applied to addition of nutrients to foods, beyond the levels originally present.

Enteral Nutrition. Tube feeding with liquid diet into stomach or intestinal tract.

Enterogastrone. An hormone which is found in the small intestine which inhibits both motor and secretory activity of the stomach. Its secretion is stimulated by fat; hence, fat in the diet inhibits gastric activity.

Enterokinase. Refers to an ingredient of the intestinal juice which activated the trypsinogen and chymotrypsinogen of the pancreatic juice to form trypsin and chymotrypsin, the active enzymes.

Entoleter. A machine which is used to disinfects cereals and other foods. The material is fed to the centre of a high-sped rotating disc carrying studs so that it is thrown against the studs and the impact kills and insects and destroys their eggs.

Enzyme. A protein catalyst. Small amounts of enzymes are able to speed up chemical reaction in cells often by many thousands of times. Each enzyme acts on a different compound and each cell contains many thousands of enzymes. There are several groups of enzymes such as the synthetases, the oxidoreductases the isomerases and the hydrolases.

Enzyme Activation Tests. Used for the diagnosis of malnutrition for vitamins (B_1, B_2, and B_6) which function as coenzymes (prosthetic groups).

The enzymes that can be so used exist in vivo as a mixture of the (inactive) apoenzyme and the (active) holoenzyme. When body reserves of the vitamin are low, the coenzyme is present in inadequate amounts. Testing the system before and after adding extra vitamin to the reaction mixture (activation) indicates whether the original levels are abnormally low. In adequately nourished subjects there can be up to 20% activation after adding the vitamin; greater stimulation is indicative of malnutrition.

Test can be performed on red blood cells for thiamin (transketolase), riboflavin (glutathione reductase) and vitamin B (aspartate or alanine aminotransferase).

Enzyme Activators. A number of small molecules can increase the activity of enzymes-these may be substrates, precursors or coenzymes such as adenine nucleotides and nicotinamide nucleotides or mineral salts, especially Ca, Mg, Cu, Mo, Zn, etc.

Enzyme, Allosteric. An enzyme which consists of multiple protein subunits can show allosteric kinetics—a change in the affinity for its substrate, and, hence, in the activity observed, as a result of changes in configuration in response to the binding of either substrates or other small molecules collectively known as allosteric effectors (they may be either activators of inhibitors).

Enzyme Induction. Refers to the synthesis of new enzyme protein in response to some stimulus such as a hormone or a substrate (e.g., drug or food additive).

Enzyme Inhibition. Many compounds are able to inhibit enzymes. Reversible inhibition is common with a number of physiological compounds, including products of the reaction or pathway, and coenzymes such as adenine and nicotinamide nucleotides. Inhibition by non-physiological compounds (drugs, food additives, etc.) may be reversible or irreversible; reversible inhibition may be competitive with respect to substrate, non-competitive or uncompetitive.

Enzyme Repression. Refers to the reduction in synthesis of enzyme protein in response to some stimulus such as a hormone or the presence of large amounts of the end-product of a pathway.

Enzyme Tenderizing. The use of proteolytic enzymes to tenderize tough meat by breaking down the structure of meat proteins. Arterial injection and multiple-needle injection are two methods of using enzymes such as papain, bromelain and ficin.

Enzymic Browing. A number of processes in which oxidoreductase enzymes present in plant tissues, e.g., phenolases, catalyse the formation of brown pigments. The substrates for these enzymes are natural compounds in the food and oxygen. The process usually spoils the food and reduces its eye appeal. Enzymic browing can be inhibited by cooking or blanching the food so that the enzymes are denatured and are no longer active or by removing oxygen, e.g., by vacuum packing, or adding chemicals which react with oxygen.

Epoxy. Prefix denoting an oxygen atom attached to two different atoms in a molecule.

Epson Salts. Magnesium sulphate; acts as a purgative because the osmotic pressure of the solution make it to retain water in the intestine and so increase the bulk of the faeces.

Equilibrium Humidity. Refers to the relative humidity of the atmosphere with which the substance under consideration is in equilibrium.

Erepsin. Name assigned to a mixture of enzymes present in the intestinal juice, including aminopeptidases and dipeptidases.

Ergosterol. Sterol isolated from yeast; when it is treated with ultraviolet light, its gets converted to vitamin D (ergocalciferol).

This is the method of manufacture of the vitamin.

Ergot. Fungus that grows on grasses and cerecal grains; the ergot of medical importance is Claviceps purpurea the grows on rye.

The consumption of infected rye is harmful, bringing about the disease known as St. Anthony's, Fire, and can be fatal.

The active principles in ergot include alkaloids, ergotinine, ergotoxine, ergotamine, ergometrine, etc. Hydrolysis of all of these produces lysergic acid, which is therefore believed to be the active component. Its effect is to increase tone and contraction of smooth muscle, especially of the pregnant uterus. For this reason ergot is used in obstetrics, but pure ergonovine maleate and ergotonine tartrate are preferable.

Ergothioneine. Betaine of thiolhistidine. It occurs in red blood cells, liver and kidney, and is constituent of ergot.

Ergotism. Refers to poisoning which occurs due to a mould infection of rye. Occurs from time to time among peoples eating rye bread.

Eriodictin. Vitamin P.

Erucic Acid. Cis-13-docosenoic acid (22-carbon monounsaturated fatty acid) occurring in Brassica napus (rape seed) and B. junca and B. nigra (mustard seed). Can constitute 30-50% of the oil in some varieties. Causes fatty infiltration of heart muscle in experimental animal among other changes, and the amount of hardened rape seed oil used n margarines is consequently limited (EEC suggested maximum is 5%; Sweden 2%).

Erythorbic Acid. D-isomer of ascorbic acid having only slight antiscorbutic activity; also called D-araboascorbic acid. Slight biological effect—May be only be protecting the vitamin C—nut it is as powerful an antioxidant as vitamin C and used in foods for that purpose.

Erythroamylose. An earlier name for amylopectin.

Erythrocytes. Red blood cells.

Erythropoiesis. Development of the red blood cells; occurs in the bone marrow.

Erythrosine BS. Red colour allowed in foods in most countries. Disodium or potassium salt of 2, 4, 5, 7-tetraiodofluorescein. It finds use in preserved cherries, sausage and meat and fish pastes; unstable to light and heat.

Escalopes. Thin pieces of meat and fish.

Esculin. Aesculin.

Essential Amino Acid Index. Protein quality.

Essential Amino Acid Pattern, Provisional. The quantities of the essential amino acids considered desirable in the diet.

Essential Amino Acids. There are 8 essential amino-acids which must be supplied by proteins in the diet as they cannot be made from any other food in the body. These essential amino acids are lysine, methionine, valine, tryptophan, leucine, isoleucine threonine and phenylalanine. Arginine and histidine may be needed for growth in children. Some protein have a balanced content of the essential amino acids and are therefore said to have a high biological value. Examples of such proteins are found in eggs, dairy products fish and meat. Proteins with a low biological value contain a less balanced content of essential amino acids, e.g. collagen (which contains only small quantities of histidine and no tryptophan and some plant proteins).

Essential Fatty Acid. Name originally assigned to linoleic acid (18C : 2 double bonds), linolenic acid (18C : 3 double bonds) and arachidonic acid (20C : 4 double bonds), found to be essential in the diets of experimental animals. Later found that only linoleic acid is essential, because it serves as a precursor for the other two although all there have a physiological role.

From the limited evidence available from human observations and animal studies the minimum requirement for linoleic acid appears to be about 1% of the total energy intake-equivalent to about 260mg per MJ; optimal intake stated to be 3-4% of energy intake (about 10g per day). Deficiency in infants gives rise to eczema; dry, thickened and scaly skin with oozing into body folds; changes in hard texture. Deficiency is very rare and there have been few reports in adolescents and adults on extremely low fat diets.

Linoleic and linolenic acids occurs in many vegetable oils (safflower, sunflower, soybean, etc.); arachidonic is found in animal fats; once termed vitamin F.

Essential Oils. Volatile, odorous oil occurring in plants. They bear no relation to the edible oils, since they are not glycerol esters. They are inflammable, soluble in alcohol and ether but not water, used for flavouring foods. Examples include oil of spearmint, oil of bitter almonds, oil of citronella, spirits of turpentine.

Ester. Chemical name of compound of acid and alcohol, e.g. ethyl alcohol and acetic aid yield ethyl acetate-an ester. Fats are esters of the trihydric alcohol glycerol, and longchain acids such as stearic or oleic.

Esterases. Name assigned to a group of enzymes tnat attack simple esters rather than fats; may be of low specificity as esterase itself, which attacks all simple esters, or of more specific nature, such as cholinesterase.

Ester Value. Same as saponification value.

Ethanolamine. 2-aminoethanol; $HOCH_2CH_2NH_2$. It occurs in plant and animal tissues as component of phospholipids; intermediate in catecholamine and phospholipid metabolism. It finds use as softening agent for hides, as dispersing agent for agricultural chemicals and as paring (peeling) agent for fruits and vegetables.

Ethanol. Systematic chemical name for ethyl alcohol.

Ethyl Alcohol. Under alcohol.

Ethylene. Refers to a gas of the formula CH_2CH_2. It is of interest in its use to assist the ripening of fruits: *e.g.* 0.4% accelerates the ripening of pears; 0.05% will convert lemons to yellow in one week at 30-40 C.

Etylene Diaminetetra-acetic Acid. Also called versene and sequestrol; forms a stable complex with metal ions and so removes them from activity.

Ethyl Formate. $HCOOC_2H_5$.

Fumigant– Used against raisin moth, dried fruit beetle, fig moth, etc.

Flavour– Ingredient of lemon and strawberry flavour and artificial run and arrack.

Chemical intermediate– In synthesis of vitamin B, sulphadiazine, etc.

Euglobulin. The name assigned to that fraction of serum globulin which gets precipitated by dialysis of blood serum against distilled water. The name implies that this fraction is a typical globulin by reason of its insolubility in water.

Euler's Yeast Coenzyme. Nicotinamide adenine dinucleotide.

Eutetic Ice. Refers to the solid which is formed when a mixture of 76.7% water and 22.3% salt (by weight) is frozen. It meals at-21°C; 3lb eutectic ice has the refrigeration effect equivalent to 1lb solid carbon dioxide; particularly useful in icing fish on board trawlers.

Eutrophia. Normal nutrition.

Evaporated Milk. The concentrated milk. Evaporated milks have no added sugar.

Evaporation, Flash. Refers to a short, rapid application of heat so that a small volume (about 1%) quickly gets distilled off carrying with it the greater part of the volatilies. The flash distillate is collected separately from the later distillate and added back to the concentrate to restore the flavour; applied to products such as fruit juices.

Evian Water. Non-gaseous, slightly mineralised; diurelic.

Exergonic. Energy-supplying reaction, such as oxidation of foodstuffs.

Exopeptidases. Enzymes that are able to split peptide bonds near the terminal units, i.e. at the ends of the protein chain. According to the older nomenclature, they were peptidases, such as aminopeptidase, carboxypeptidase and dipeptidases of the digestive juices.

Exotoxins. Refers to the toxic substances which are produced by bacteria and diffuse out of the cells; stimulate antibodies which specifically neutralise them; generally heat-labile and inactivated in 1 hour at 60°C. Exotoxins include those produced by botulism, tetanus and diphtheria organisms.

Expansing Ring. In relation to cans, this term is used to refer to the concentric rings stamped into the ends of the can to allow bulging during heat processing without staining the seams unduly.

Expeller Cake. Oilseed after removal of most of the oil by pressing; a valuable source of protein. (Cotton, coconut, groundnut sunflower, sesame, etc.)

Extensograph. An instrument which is used for measuring the stretching quality of a dough as an index of its backing quality; the dough is stretched in cylindrical form.

Extensometer. An instrument which is used to measure the stretching strength of a dough as an index of its backing quality. A ball of fermenting dough is fixed on two pins which are moved apart to stretch the dough.

Extraction. The process of removing a substance or mixture of substances from a food. Extraction can also mean the removal of a part of a food, e.g. the extraction of juice from fruits such as oranges.

Extraction Rate. Refers to the yield of flour which is obtained from wheat in the milling process. 100% extraction (or straight-run flour) is wholemeal flour containing all of the grain; lower extraction rates are the whiter flours from which more of the bran and the germ are excluded, down to a figure of 72% extraction, white is the normal which flour of commerce.

'Patent' flours have been of lower extraction rate, 30-50g, and so comprise mostly the endosperm of the grain.

Analysis per 10g : 72g extraction : protein 8-12.5g, fibre 0.1-0.2, vitamin B 0.1mg, vitamin B 0.06mg, nicotinic acid 0.8mg, Fe 1.5mg.

80% extraction : protein 9-12.5g, fibre 0.2-0.3 g, vitamin B 0.25mg, vitamin B 0.07mg, nicotinic acid 1.6mg, Fe 1.7mg.

100% extraction (wholemeal) : protein 10-14g, fibre 1.5-2.0g, vitamin B 0.4mg, vitamin B 0.3mg, nicotinic acid 5.5mg, fe 3.0mg.

F

Facultative Aerobes. Bacteria which grow best in the presence of oxygen but can grow anaerobically.

Facultative Anaerobes. Bacteria which grow best in the absence of oxygen but can grow aerobically.

FAD. Flavine adenine dinucleotide.

Faeces. Refers to the composition of undigested food residues, remains of digestive secretions not reabsorbed, bacteria from the intestinal lining, substances excreted into the intestinal tract. Average 100g intestinal tract, cells and mucus from the intestinal lining, substances excreted into the intestinal tract. Average 100g per day. Principal pigment, stercobilin.

Faggot.

1. Refers to the small bundle of parsley, thyme, marjoram and bay leaf tied together with cotton and added to the dish being cooked. Also known as bouquet garni.
2. Dish of liver, chopped, seasoned and baked.

FAO. Food and Agriculture Organization of the United Nations.

Farex. Trade name (Glaxo Laboratories) of an infant cereal food. Analysis per 100g : protein 12.9g, fat 2.3g, carbohydrate 73g, Ca 885mg, Fe 24mg, keal 348 (1.4 MJ), vitamin B_1 1.4mg, vitamin B_2 1.6mg.

Farina. General term for starch. More specifically it refers to potato starch; but in some countries it is defined as the starch obtained from wheat other than durum wheat, starch from the later is semolina.

Farina Dolce. Italian flour which is made from dried chestnuts.

Farinograph. An instrument used to measure the stability and consistency of dough. The machine measures the force needed to turn a set of blades at a set speed in a dough mixture.

Farlene. A trade name (Farley's Infant Food, Plymouth) for a high protein baby food in the form of a dried powder. It is composed of wheat flour, high-protein wheat flour, soya, peas, milk, wheat gluten and egg, fortified with vitamins and minerals.

Analysis per 100g : Protein 25g. fat 5.5g, carbohydrate 61.5g, kcal 390 (1.6MJ), Ca 0.8g, Fe 12mg, vitamin A 840µg, vitamin B 0.8mg, vitamin B 0.6mg, nicotinic acid 15mg, vitamin C 70mg, vitamin D 18µg.

Fast Foods. A general term which is used for a limited menu of foods that lend themselves to production line techniques; suppliers tend to specialise in products such as hamburgers, pizzas, chicken or sandwiches.

Fat Blood. About 590mg per 100ml plasma; 150mg neutral fat 160mg cholesterol, 200mg phospholipid.

Fat-extenders. Refers to substances that allow a reduction of fat content without altering the texture, used in baked products, e. g., glyceryl monostearate.

Fatfold Test. A test of body fatness by measuring the thickness of a fold of skin on the arm back or other part of the body.

Fat, Netural. Refers to the triglyceride fats. It is used in distinction from other lipids, as, for example, in blood, where the subdivision is neutral fat, cholesterol and phospholipid.

Fats.

1. Chemically fats are defined as substances which are insoluble in water but soluble in organic solvent such as ether, chloroform and benzene, and are actual or potential esters of fatty acid. The term includes triglycerides, phospholipids, waxes and sterols; also

termed lipids.

2. In the more general use the term 'fats' refers to the netural fats which are mixtures of esters of fatty acids with glycerol i.e. triglycerides.

Fats, High-ratio. Refers to the shortening with a greater proportion of mono and diglycerides, i.e. superglycerinated (also superglycinerated fats.) These shortenings disperse more readily into doughs, and allow the use of a higher ratio of sugar to flour than with ordinary shortening.

Fats, Hydrogenated. Hydrogenated oils.

Fat-soluble Vitamins. Vitamins A, D, E and K. These are found in food in solution in the fasts. Are stored in the body to a greater extent than the water-soluble.

Fatty Acids. Organic acids which are consisting of carbon chains with a carboxyl group at the end. Simplest is formic acid, HCOOH then acetic acid, CH_3COOH propionic butyric etc.

Longer-chain fatty acids include those found in soap, like stearic, palmitic and oleic.

They may be saturated fatty acids, in which every carbon atom carried its full quota of hydrogen atoms, or unsaturated, in which there is a shortage of hydrogen atoms compensated for by a double instead of a single bond linking two adjacent carbon atoms. Such double bonds are susceptible to the addition of oxygen and, hence, unsaturated fatty acids (and unsaturated fats made from them) are less stable than fully saturated ones. Fats with a large number of double bonds, i.e. highly unsaturated, readily oxidise to resin-like consistency and are the so-called 'drying oils' such as linseed and tung oil, used in paints.

Fatty Acids, Essential. Essential fatty acids.

Fatty Acids, Free

1. Liberated from triglycerides when subjected to hydrolytic rancidity; therefore determination of FFA is an index of quality of fats.

2. Also non-esterified fatty acids.

Fecula. Name assigned to foods which are almost solely starch; prepared from roots and stems by grating, e.g. tapioca, sago and arrowroot.

Favisum. Acute haemolytic anaemia which is induced in genetically sensitive people by eating broad beans, Vicia faba. The genetic disease refers to a deficiency of the enzyme glucose-6-phosphate dehydrogenase in the red blood cells, which are usually vulnerable to the toxins, vicine and convincine, in the beans.

Fehling's Solution. Fehling's test.

Fehling's Test. For reducing substances, mostly used for distinguishing reducing from non-reducing sugars. Depends upon the reduction of blue cupric hydroxide to yellow cuprous oxide on heating the alkaline solution. Fehling's solution A is copper sulphate, and solution B is alkaline tartrate; mixed immediately before use to prevent deterioration.

Fennel. Foeniculum vulgare (Parsely family): sees have 10% fixed oil and 6% essential oil, containing anethole, fenchone and terpenes. Leaves used in fish dishes and sauces.

Fenugreek. Trigonella feonumgraecum. Leguminous plant eaten as vegetable, seeds used for flovouring. Consumed by women in Orient to help gain weight.

Analysis of seeds per 100g : 29g protein, 5g fat, 50g carbohydrate, 355 kcal (1.46MJ), 180mg Ca, 22mg Fe, 0.4mg vitamin B, 0.3mg vitamin B, 1.5mg nicotinic acid.

Ferguzade. A trade name (Ferguzade Ltd) for a glucose beverage.

Ferment. As a noun, the old name for enzyme. As a verb, to carry out the process of fermentation.

Fermentation. Anaerobic metabolism. Used generally of alcohol fermentation of sugars, also production of latic acid, citric acid, etc., by micro-organisms.

Fermented Milk. Milks, fermented.

Fermentograph. An instrument which is used for measuring the gas-producing power of a dough. The fermenting dough is contained in a balloon immersed in water and as gas is produced the balloon expands and rises in the water, the rise being measured continuously.

Ferric Ammonium Citrate. Refers to the form in which iron is sometimes added to foods. It is found as brown-red scales (16.5-18.5% iron) and as green scales (14.5-16% iron).

Ferritin. Refers to a ferric hydroxide-phosphate-protein complex (containing 23% iron) which is present in the cells of the intestinal mucosa, liver, spleen and bone marrow, as a storage form of iron.

Ferrum Redactum. Iron, reduced.

FFA. Free fatty acids.

Fibre, Crude. Term given to indigestible part of foods, defined as the residue left after successive extractions with petroleum ether, 1.25% sulphuric acid and 1.25% sodium hydroxide minus ash, carried out under closely specified conditions. Dietary fibre bears no real relation to crude fibre and its estimation involves a series of specified procedures.

Fibre, Dietary. Collective term for the structural parts of plant tissues which are not digested (or only part-digested) by man and include cellulose, hemicelluloses, lignin, pectins and gums. They are of varying composition and have a range of physicochemical and physiological properties. It is the modern term for what was previously variously called roughage or bulk.

Dietary fibre has been not the same as crude fibre, which see, and in many cereal foods the content of dietary fibre is greater than that of crude fibre.

Fibrin

1. Fibrinogen.
2. Discarded name for one of the muscle proteins, once called 'albumin' and 'fibrin'.

Fibrinogen. Refers to one of the proteins of the blood plasma which is responsible for the clotting of blood. Under the influence of thrombin it is converted to fibrin, which is deposited as strands that trap the red cells and form the clot.

Fibrous Proteins. Albuminoids.

Ficin. Proteolytic enzyme from the fig.

Fig. Ficus carica; eaten fresh, dried (when they are having 50% sugars) and preserved; have mild laxative properties, e.g. syrup of figs is a medicinal preparation. Analysis per 10g : 13g protein 11g carbohydrate, 49 kcal (0.2MJ), 1mg Fe, 24μg vitamin A 0.1mg vitamin B_1, 0.08mg vitamin B_2, 17mg nicotinic acid, zero vitamin C. Dried figs : 4g protein, 63g carbohydrate, 262 kcal (1.1MJ), 200mg Ca, 4mg Fe, 30μg vitamin A, 0.1mg vitamin B_1, 0.08mg vitamin B_2, 1.7mg nicotinic acid, Zero vitamin C.

FIGLU Test. Formiminoglutamic acid, test.

Filix Mas. Male fern; having organic acids, including filicic acid, which have a selective action on, and therefore used in treatment for, tapeworm.

Filled Milk. A dehydrated milk made from skim milk to which vegetable oil has been added before the product is dried. Various level of oil can be added depending on the intended use. Filled milk has a much better shelf-life than dried whole milk.

Film Yeasts. Yeast.

Filth Test. Name assigned to a test originated in the USA for determining the contamination of a food with rodent hairs and insect fragment as an index of the hygienic handing of the food.

Filtrate Factor. Pantothenic acid.

Fines Herbes. Refers to a mixture of chopped parsley, chervil, chives and tarragon.

Fining Agents. Refers to substances which are used to clarify liquids by precipitating and carrying down suspended matter, e.g. egg albumin, casein, bentonite, isinglass, gelatin, etc.

Finnan Haddock. Smoke-cured haddock.

Fireless Cooker. Haybox.

Fire Point. With reference to frying oils it refers to the temperature at which the fat will sustain combustion. It ranges between 340° and 360°C for different fats.

Firkin. Refers to a quarter of a barrel of beer, i.e. 9 imperial gallons; also 56lb of butter.

Firming Agents. Fresh fruits are having insoluble pectins as a firm gel around the fibrous tissues and keep the fruit firm. Break down of cell structure permits conversion of pectin to pectin acid, with loss of firmness. Addition of calcium salts (chloride or carbonate) yields calcium pectate gel which protects the fruit against softening; these are known as firming agents.

Alum is sometimes used to firm pickles.

Fish. The composition of all non-fatty fish, such as cod, hake, had dock, flatfish, is similar.

Fish, Fatty. Anchovies, herring, mackerel, salmon, sardines-having about 15% fat (varying from 5 to 20% throughout the year) and containing 10-14gu vitamin D per 10g, as distinct from white fish, which contain 1-2% fat and only a trace of vitamin D.

Fish Ham. Japanese product which is obtained from a red fish such as tuna or marlin, pickled with salt and nitrite, mixed with whale meat and pork fat and stuffed into a large sausage-type casing.

Fish Meal. Surplus fish, waste from filleting (fish-house waste) and fish unfit for human consumption are dried in vacuum, by steam, or hot air, and powdered.

The resultant fish meal has been a valuable source of protein as animal feedingstuff, or, after deodorisation, as human food, since it contain about 70% protein of biological value up to 75.

That made from white fish is termed white fish meal, as distinct form the oily type. The latter is sometimes of very poor quality and then finds use as fertiliser.

Fish Paste. A spread which is made from ground fish and cereal.

Fish Protein Concentrate. Deodorised, decolorised, defatted fish meal also known as fish flour. Cheap source of protein for enrichment of foods.

Approximately it is 75% protein; and its biological value is 75-80.

Fish Sausage. A Japanese product which is made from chopped fish fillet, spiced, flavoured, plus fat and starch, and the whole packed into sausage casing.

Fistula. A short-circuiting connection. For example, an Eck fistula is a surgical joining of the portal vein to the inferior vena cava, so that the liver is short-circuited. Used as an experimental technique for examining the function of the liver.

Flamber. To light spirit poured over a dish, e.g. brandy on the Christmas pudding.

Flash Evaporation. Evaporation, flash.

Flash-pasteurisation. Refers to the process in which the material is held at a higher temperature than in normal pasteurisation, but for a shorter period. There is less development of the cooked flavour in the shorter period. For milk, ordinary pasteurisation involved heating to 60°C for 33 seconds; in the flash process 74°C for only a few seconds.

Flash Point. With reference to frying oils, it refers to the temperature at which the decomposition products can be ignited, but will not support combustion. Whey they will support combustion, this is the fire point. Cottonseed oil : smoke points 232°C. These points are lowered by the presence of free fatty acids.

Flash point gets varied with different fast, and ranges between 290° and 330°C.

Flash 18. Refers to a method of canning foods under pressure 18 pounds per square inch above atmospheric pressure. The food is sterilised at 121°C and then canned at that temperature, not requiring further heat.

The advantages claimed include improved taste and texture compared with conventional canning, and the possibility of using large container without overheating the food.

Flatogens. Refers to the substance that causes gas production, flatulence in the intestine. Those identified include raffinose, stachyose and verbascose in a variety of beans

Flat Sours. Refers to the Bacteria that render canned food sour, without gas production, i.e. the ends of the can are not swelled out but remain flat. They have been thermophilic, facultative anaerobes, which attack carbohydrates with the production of acids, lactic, formic acetic, but without gas formation.

Economically they are the most important of the thermophilic spilage agents, some species can grow slowly at 25°C and therefore spoil products after long storage periods. Type species is Bacillus stearothermophilus.

Flatulence. Refers to the production of gas in the intestine-hydrogen, carbon dioxide and methane. It is possibly caused by a variety of foods, including beans, Brussels sprouts cabbage, cauliflower, onions, radishes, melon, avocado, which contain indigestible carbohydrates which are fermented by the bacteria in the intestine.

Flatus. Gas production in the intestinal tract, which arises either from the stomach (released by mouth) or the colon (released rectally). Undigested sugars (stachyose, raffinose and verbascose) serve as substrate for intestinal bacteria, with the production of methane, carbon dioxide and hydrogen.

Flavedo. Refers to the coloured outer peel layer of citrus fruits. It is also called the epicarp or zest. It contains the oil sacs and numerous yellow plastics (green in the unripe fruit, containing chlorophyll; yellow in the ripe fruit, containing carotene and xanthophyll).

Flavin. Also called quercitron. A colour which is obtained from the quercitron bark (species of oak, Quercus tinctoria); legally permitted in food in most countries. It is insoluble in water but soluble in alkalies to give yellow colour, changed to brown in air.

Flavin Adenine Dinucleotide (FAD). Coenzyme in cellular oxidation having the vitamin riboflavin, attached to two phosphate molecules, and ribose and adenine.

Flavins. Derivatives of iso-alloxazine, as in riboflavin (the

6,7 dimethyl derivative).

Flavone. Flavonoids.

Flavonoids. Compounds which are widely distributed in nature as pigments in flowers, fruit, vegetables and tree barks.

Structurally the flavone nucleus is having a benzenoid ring which is fused to gamma-pyrone carrying a second benzenoid ring and bearing a number of hydroxyl groups. Flavonoids are flavone glycosides with rhamnose or rhamnoglucose attached at position 3 or 7.

Flavonoids are divided into flavonols-hydroxy; group replaces H in flavone nucleus; flavanone-one double bond reduced in the 2 = 3 position; flavonols-hydroxyl group in place of the O and reduction of double bond at 4 and reduction of 2 = 3 double bond; isoflavones-benzenoid ring attached to C_3 instead of C_2.

Flavonols. Flavonoids.

Flavoproteins. Refers to a group of oxidising enzymes which are composed of conjugated proteins containing riboflavin (vitamin B_2) as the prosthetic group. There are two classes, those containing flavin mononucleotide, and those containing adenineflavin dinucleotide. The protein itself differs in each specific enzyme.

Examples: Amino acid oxidase (which oxidises amino acids to ketonic acids), cytochrome reductase (part of the oxidation chain in the cell), diaphorase and Warburg'g yellow enzyme (also part of the oxidation chain).

Flavour. Organoleptic.

Flavour Potentiator Refers to as substance that enhances the flavours of other substance without itself imparting any characteristic flavour of its own, e.g., monosodium glutamate, ribotide, as well as small quantities of sugar, salt and vinegar.

Flavour Profile. Refers to a method or judging flavour of foods by examination of a list of the separate factors into which the flavour can be analysed-the so-called character notes.

Flavours, Synthetic. Mostly mixtures of esters, e.g. banana oil ethyl butyrate and amyl acetate; apple oil-ethyl butyrate, ethyl valerianate, ethyl salicylate, amyl butyrate, glycerol, chloroform and alcohol; pineapple oil-ethyl and amyl butyrates, a acetal dehyde, chloroform, glycerol, alcohol.

Flipper. Swells.

Florenec Oil. Name assigned to high grade of olive oil.

Floridean Starch. A glucosan which is resembling glycogen and obtained from red algae (Florideae).

Flour. Generally refers to the ground wheat berry, although also used for other cereals and applied to powdered dried materials like fish flour (deodorised dried fish), potato flour etc.

The ground wheat berry yields wholemeal, flour (100% extraction); whiter flours are obtained by separation of the bran and the germ from the starchy endosperm.

The white flour as used in the ordinary white loaf is 70-72% extraction fortified to contain not less than 0.24 mg vitamin B^1 1.6mg nicotinic acid, and 1.65mg iron per 100g plus 140z of Creta Praeparata (chalk) per 280lb sack of flour.

Flour Enrichment. Refers to the addition of certain vitamins and minerals to flour.

Flour, High-ratio. Refers to flour of very fine and more uniform particle size, treated with chlorine to reduce the gluten strength. Used for making cakes, since it is possible to add up to 140 parts of sugar to 100 parts of this flour, whereas only half this quantity of sugar can be incorporated into cakes with ordinary flour.

Flour, Self-raising. Refers to the flour to which have been added chemicals that produce carbon dioxide in the presence of water and heat; the dough is thus aerated without prolonged fermentation. Usually 'weaker' flours are used.

Chemical agents used: sodium carbonate (3lb 40z per 280lb sack); calcium acid phosphate or sodium pyrophosphate (41/3 lb); or a mixture of these two.

Legally, self-rasing flour must contain not less than 0.4% available carbon dioxide.

Flour Strength. Refers to a property of the flour proteins enabling the dough to retain gas during fermentation to give a 'bold' loaf, 'strong' flour is higher in protein content, has greater elasticity and resistance to extension, and greater ability to absorb water. A 'weak' flour give a loaf that lacks volume.

Fluid Bed Dryer. A bed of solid particles is supported on a cushion of hot air jets (fluidised) and the material may be conveyed in this way, while being dried. The method achieves intimate mixing without mechanical damage : it is applicable to particles of a size sufficiently small to become impervious when packed closely and sufficiently large to float on an air cushions (as distinct from fine powders), e.g., cereals, tabletting granules, salt, coffee and dried vegetables.

Flummery. Another name for frumenty.

Fluorscence. Refers to the ability to absorb light at one wavelength and radiate part of it at another wavelength. It finds use analytically for quantitative measurement by fluorimetry, the intensity of fluorescence being proportional to the amount of material present. For example, vitamin B_2 and thiochrome, prepared from vitamin B fluoresce.

Fluoridation. Fluorine.

Fluorimetry. Fluorescence.

Fluorine. An element of the same family as chlorine, bromine and iodine (the halogens). It ordinarily occurs in small amounts in plants and animals.

Drinking water ranges in fluoride content between 0.05 and 14 parts per million, and water containing concentrations around 1ppm helps to protect teeth from decay, although the mechanism of this effect is unknown. Quantities of this order are added to drinking water in enlightened areas to confer this protection. In larger amounts it brings about chalky white patches to appear on the surface of the teeth, known as mottled enamel.

Excessive doses are toxic and give rise to fluorosis.

FMN. Flavine mononucleotide.

Foam-mat Drying. Refers to a method of drying food. The liquid concentrate is whipped to a foam white the aid of a foaming agent, spread on a tray and dried in a stream of warm air. It reconstitutes very rapidly with water because of the fine structure of the foam. It has the further advantage that the foam dried materials hold less water at a given relative humidity than do spray-dried foods and are less liable to cake.

Folic Acid. Or folocin. A vitamin: generic descriptor for a group of substances which are essential for the synthesis of purines and pyrimidines and so for nucleic acid synthesis, and all processes of cell division. Functions by serving as a carrier of one-carbon units: deficiency signs include megaloblastic anaemia.

The active principle has been tetrahydrofolic acid or folinic acid (tetrahydropteroyl glutamic acid). The numerous chemical derivatives five rise to various names over the years of their elucidation-citrovorum factor (CF) and leucovorin (5-formyl tetrahydroglutamic acid), rhizopterin, SLR (streptococcus lactis R) factor, Wills factor, vitamin M, vitamin B_1, factors U, R and S-all of which consist of pteroyl glutamic acid with up to six additional glutamyl residues.

It occurs in liver, kidneys, green leafy vegetable and yeast.

Fondant. Minute sugar crystals in a saturated sugar syrup. It is used as the creamy filling in chocolates and biscuits and for decorating cakes. Prepared by boiling sugar solution with addition of confectioners' glucose or an inverting agent and cooling rapidly while stirring.

Food. Substances which are taken in by mouth which maintain life and growth, i.e., supply energy, and build and replace tissue.

Food Allergy. An unusually bodily response in person to a food or foods that do not produce a response in most people. Many effects or symptoms have been described in people sensitive to foods allergens including disorders of the alimentary canal skin and lungs. Other symptoms, including hyperactivity in children, have been reported but are not so well understood.

Food Analogue. A food made to appear, smell, feel and taste the same as a natural food. Food analogues are fabricated foods, e.g., margarine, meat analogue made from textured vegetable protein.

Food Phosphate Factor. May be defined as the ration between the resistance to heat when present in a food and the resistance when in phosphate buffer (at pH 6.98). The protective action of the ingredients of food renders the bacteria more resistant than in buffer.

Food Poisoning. May occur due to (1) contamination with harmful bacteria; (2) toxic chemicals; (3) allergic reaction to certain proteins; (4) chemical contamination.

The commonest bacterial contamination has been due to salmonella, staphylococci and Clostridium welchil. Staphylococcal poisoning causes rapid symptoms within 2-4 hours of abdominal cramp, nausea, vomiting and diarrhoea; recovery is rapid.

Salmonellae gives rise to an endotoxin which is not destroyed by cooking and causes acute gastroenteritis after 12-24 hours. It is not often fatal but nausea, vomiting and diarrhoea may persist several weeks.

Very rarely food poisoning occurs die to Clostridium botulinum. i.e. botulism, where see.

Food Scientist. Refers to one who studied the basic chemical and physical, biochemical and biophysical properties of foods and their constituents.

Food Spoilage. Any damage caused to food which does not necessarily make it harmful but makes it inedible. There are three kinds of food spoilage; enzymic browning, autolysis and microbiological spoilage.

Food Technologist. Refers to one who applies food science to the preservation, processing and preparation of foods, and to their packaging, storage and transportation.

Force. The name for a breakfast cereal which is made from wheat flakes. Not fortified with added vitamins; natural content 0.07mg vitamin B_1 and 0.07MG vitamin B_2 per 100mg.

Forcemeat. Refers to a highly seasoned stuffing which is made from chopped or minced veal or pork or sausage meat mixed with onion and a range of herbs (form French, force, stuffing).

Formiminoglutamic Acid Test (FIGLU).. Test for vitamin B_{12} deficiency which is based on the enhanced excretion of formiminoglutamic acid in the urine following a test dose of histidine.

Formula 21. 'Slimming' preparation which is composed of methyl cellulose and glucose, with flavour and colour, plus vitamin B 1.1mg, vitamin B_2 2.7mg, nicotinic acid 10.9mg, reduced iron 10.9mg, Ca 675mg per oz.

Fortifex. Protein-rich baby food (30% protein) developed in Brazil; made from maize, defatted soya flour with added vitamins A, B_1, B_2, calcium carbonate and methionine.

FPC. Fish protein concentrate.

Fractional Test Meal. Method of examining secretion of gastric juices of patients. The stomach contents are sampled at intervals via a stomach tube after a test meal or gruel. It is usual to test for total and free acidity, and in addition peptic activity may be measured.

Fragmentation-milling. A kind of roller-milling in which the white flour is further divided into three groups of particle size using a stream of air.

Frangipane. Originally a jasmine perfume, which gave its name to an almond cream flavoured with the perfume. The term is used for cake-filling made from eggs, milk and flour with flavouring, and also for the pastry filled with an almond-flavoured mixture.

Frappe. Egg-white and sugar syrup whipped until so aerated that the density reaches 5lb gallon.

Frederickson's Classification. Refers to a system of classifying hyperlipidaemias according to types of plasma lipoproteins which are elevated.

Freeze Concentration. Refers to the concentration of a liquid by freezing out pure ice, leaving a more concentrated solution, of interest in the concentration of fruit juices, vinegar and beer.

Freeze Drying. Refers to a method of drying in which the material is frozen and subjected to high vacuum. The ice sublimes off as water vapour without melting. Materials dried in this way are damaged little, if at all. Freeze-dried food has been very porous, because it occupies the same volume as the original and so rehydrates rapidly. There is less loss of flavour and texture than with most other methods of drying. Controlled heat may be applied to the process without melting the frozen material-this is accelerated freeze drying.

Freezerburn. Refers to a change in the texture of frozen meat, fist and poultry during storage due to sublimation of the ice.

Freezing. A process in which food is preserved by being cooled to temperatures below 0°C and normally as low as -20°. The water and many of the components of food solidify during freezing. Because micro-organisms require liquid water for their life processes which normally function at higher temperature, freezing inhibits their growth. Foods such as plants are belched or cooked before freezing but meats and fish can be stored without treatment.

French Dressing. Refers to temporary emulsion of oil and acid, in distinction to mayonnaise, which is a stable emulsion. Heavy French dressing is a similar product stabilised with pectin or vegetable gum.

Frenching. Refers to the breaking up the fibres of meat by cutting, usually diagonally or in a criss-cross pattern.

Frigi-Canning. Refers to a process of preserving food by controlled heating, sufficient to destroy the vegetative form of micro-organism (and possible to damage spores sufficiently to prevent germination) followed by sealing aseptically and storing at a low temperature but not at freezing point.

Fructosan. A complex which is built up of units of fructose.

Fructose. A six-carbon sugar-$C_6H_{12}O_6$- differing from glucose in containing a ketonic group (on C_2) instead of an aldehyde group (which glucose has on C_1).

Found as the free sugar in some fruits and in honey and combined with glucose as sucrose. Prepared by the hydrolysis of insulin from the Jerusalem artichoke. Alternative names fruit sugar and laevulose; 173% as sweet as sucrose.

Fructose rotates polarised light to the left (hence the name laevulose), in distinction from glucose, which rotates polarised light to the right.

Fructose Syrups. (high-fructose glucose syrups). Glucose syrups having more than 10% fructose produced by enzymatic or alkali conversion; can be 35% glucose, 45% fructose and 5-10% maltose, and then they are as sweet as sucrose, with viscosity similar to that of 67% sucrose solution; used in soft drinks, canned fruits, jams and preserves and bakery products; Also termed isosyrups.

Fruit. Refers to the fleshy seed-bearing part of plants (including tomato, usually called a vegetable). Contain negligible protein and fat; carbohydrate varies from 3% in melon to 25% in banana. Carbohydrate occurs as glucose, fructose, sucrose, starch, pectin and cellulose. Cellulose adds bulk to the diet, pectin give jellying power to fruit.

During repining of fruit starch changes to sugars. Fruits are a good source of potassium and vitamin C, and some are a useful source of carotene and iron.

Fruit, Canned. The fruit is usually canned in a sugar solution and, hence, the energy content is greater than that of the fresh fruit.

Analysis per 100g of, for example, fresh peaches (without stones): 9g carbohydrate, 37 kcal (0.15 MJ); condemn 17.2g carbohydrate 66 kcal (0.27 MJ).

Vitamin loss has been about 50%, e.g. peaches lose half of the carotene, vitamins B_1 and B_2 nicotinic acid and vitamin C in canning.

Fruit Cordials. Soft drinks.

Fruit, Dried. Dried figs, dates, prunes and raisins, all are having similar analyses.

Protein 2.5g, fat 0.6g, 255 kcal (1.06 MJ), Ca 73mg, Fe 2.7mg, vitamin A 20μg, vitamin B_1 0.1mg, vitamin B_2 0.1mg, nicotinic acid 1.5mg, vitamin C nil-per 100g.

Fruit Drinks. Soft drinks.

Fruit- Squash. Soft drinks.

Frumenty. Whole wheat which is stewed in water for 24 hours until the grains have burst and set in a thick jelly, then boiled with milk.

Frying. Involves rapid evaporation of water. In the case of meat nearly all the extractive are left in the meat and the losses are smaller than in roasting. About 10-20% loss of vitamin B_1, 10-15% loss of vitamin B_2 and nicotinic acid. Fish loses 20% vitamin B_1.

Fudge. Caramel in which crystallisation of the sugar (graining) gets deliberately induced by the addition of fondant (saturated syrup containing sugar crystals).

Fumeol. Refined smoke having the bitter principles removed. It is used for preparing 'liquid' smokes for dipping foods such as fish to give them a smoked flavour.

Fungal Protein. Mould mycelium.

Fungi. Sub-division of Thallophyta, plants without differentiation into root, stem and leaf; cannot photosynthesis, all are parasites or saprophytes. Varieties of Penicillium, Aspergillus, etc., have been the cause of deterioration in foods in the presence of oxygen and relative humidity of at least 70%. On the other hand, varieties of Penicillium such as P. Cambertii and P rocquefortii are desirable in certain cheeses.

Among the edible fungi include mushrooms, Agaricus campestris. Experimentally, varieties like Graphium, Fusarium, and Rhizopus are grown on waste carbohydrates as a potential food; their fibrillar structure offers textural advantages in foods manufactured from them.

Furcellaran. Danish agar. Refers to an anionic, sulphated polysaccharide extracted from the red alga, Furcellaria fastigiata, structurally similar to carrageenan; used as a galling agent.

Fusel Oil. Alcoholic fermentation produces about 95% alcohol and 5% fusel oil—a mixture of organic acids, higher alcohol (propyl, butyl and amyl), aldehydes and esters.

Present in low concentration in wines and beer and higher concentration in pt-still spirit. On maturation of the liquor the fusel oil changes and imparts the special flavour to the spirit.

Fussol. Monofluoroacetamide—a systemic insecticide which is used for treating fruit.

Fustic. Colouring matter which is obtained from the tree chlorophora tinctoria or Maclura tinctoria. Two colour agents presents, morin, sparingly, soluble in water but soluble in alcohol, and maclurin, more soluble. Both are yellow but altered by alkali and metals.

F Value. Unit of measurement which is used to compare relative sterilising effects of different procedures; equal to 1 minute at 121.1°C.

G

Galactosaemia. Refers to inherited inability to metabolise the sugar galactose beyond the formation of its phosphate.

Galactose. Refers to a six-carbon sugar which is differing from glucose only in the position of the hydroxyl group on C_4.

It occurs mainly linked with glucose to form lactose (milk sugar), and also occurs in the galactolipids of nerve tissue. Has 32% of the sweetness of sucrose.

Galantine. Refers to a dish of white meat or poultry, boned, rolled, cooked with herbs, glazed with aspic jelly and served cold.

Galenicals. Crude drugs, infusions, decoctions and tinctures which are prepared from medicinal plants.

Gallates. Salts and esters of gallic acid which are found in many plants. These find use in making dyes and inks, and medicinally as an astringent.

Gall-bladder. Organ which is situated in the liver. It stores the bile manufactured by the liver.

Gallon. Imperial gallon is 4.546 liters (=10lb of water at 17°C). US gallon is 3.7853 litres; Imperial gallon = 1.2 US gallons.

Gall-stones (cholelithiasis). Concretions which are composed of cholesterol, bile pigments and calcium salts, formed in the gallbladder or bile due when the bile becomes supersaturated.

Game. None-domesticated (*i.e.,* wild) animals and birds.

Gammon. Hind legs of bacon pig, cured while still part of carcass.

Garbenzo. Chickpea (Cicer arietinum).

Garlic. Bulb of Allium sativum (lity family) having pungent odour when crushed. This occurs due to diallyl thiosulphinate, ammonia and pyruvic acid liberated from an odourless precursor, alien (allyl-cysteine sulphoxide) by the enzyme alliinase. Diallyl disulphide derived from diallyl thiosulphinate has been responsible for the characteristic odour of garlic.

Gas Storage, Controlled. Storage of fruits and vegetable in a controlled atmosphere in which the proportion of oxygen is reduced and that of carbon dioxide increased.

Gastrin. Polypeptide hormones (I and II) secreted in stomach. These stimulate secretion of gastric HCl and pancreatic enzyme output.

Gastric Secretion. Gastric juice is having of the enzymes pepsin, renin and lipase, together with mucin and hydrochloric acid. The acid is secreted by the parietal cells at a strength of 0.16N = 0.5-0.6% acid. The pepsin is secreted by the chief cells, and the mucin by the mucous cells. Pepsin requires an acid medium of function and breaks down proteins to proteoses.

The main function of rennin is to coagulate milk. The small amount of lipase resent splits only a very small proportion of that fat.

Gastrin. Hormone which is secreted by the pyloric antrum of the stomach under the influence of certain foods (especially meat) and by distension of the stomach. The gastrin enters the blood stream and stimulates the secretion of gastric juice.

Gastro-intestical Tract. A term which is covering the whole of the digestive tract, from the mouth to the anus. Average length 4.5 meters (15 feet).

Gefillte Fish. Also spelled 'gefilte' and 'gefultte'. Literally, German for stuffed fish. The dish is of Russian or Polish origin, where it is commonly called Jewish fish. The whole fish is served and the filleted portion chopped and stuffed back between the skin and the backbone. More frequently today, the fist is simply chopped into a pulp and made into balls.

Gel. Refers to a sol or colloidal suspension that has set to a jelly.

Gelatin. Water-soluble protein which is prepared from collagen by boiling with water, or from bones. As a protein it is of poor nutritive value, since it lacks tryptophan.

Gelatin Sugar. Glycine.

Genetic Disease. In connection with food, this refers to the inherited inability to metabolise certain dietary factors, often with harmful results.

Gerber Test. Two molecules of glucose which are joined 1.6-β.

Gerber Test. Test for fat in milk. When sulphuric acid and milk are mixed, heat develops, the organic matter dissolves, but not the fat. This separates, aided by the addition of amyl alcohol. The reaction is carried out in a Gerber bottle having a thin, graduated neck, in which the fat collects, and is measured. Used for routine analyses of milk.

Germ, Wheat. Refers to the embryo or sporting portion of the wheat berry which is comprising about 2.5% of seed. Contains 64% of the thiamin, 26% of the riboflavin, 21% of the pyridoxine and most of the fat of the wheat grain, and gets discarded when the grain is milled to white flour.

Ghee. Clarified butter fat made by heating and separating the water, made from milk of cow, buffalo, goat or sheep. Widely used in India; does not go rancid as quickly as butter; Egyptian equivalent is samna.

Gherkin. Cucumis anguria. Young green cucumber of small variety, used for pickling.

Gibberellic Acid. Originally occur in the fungus Gibberella fujikuroi growing on rice. About 30 gibberelins are known; they are plant growth hormones which bring about stem extension and allow mutant dwarf forms of plants to revert to normal size, induce flower formation, break bud dormancy; used to accelerate germination of barely for brewing purposes; influence the synthesis of DNA.

Gin. Spirit having 31% alcohol flavoured with juniper berries and other flavours; 220 kcal (0.9 MJ) per 10ml. Name derived from French genievre, meaning juniper; originally know as Geneva, Schiedam and Hollands, because it is Dutch in origin.

Ginger. Rhizome of zingiber officinale. It is used as a flavouring; pungency due to non-volatile compounds, including gingerol, zingerone and shogool.

Glasgow Magistrate. Term for red herring.

Gliadin. Refers to one of the proteins of wheat; gliadin and glutenin compose what is generally called gluten, the protein mixture which forms the basis of dough formation. Gliadin is the protein responsible for coelic disease.

Globins. Basic proteins that differ from histones, because they are rich in histidine, deficient in isoleucine and contain average amounts of arginine and tryptophan. Globins are simple proteins themselves (*i.e.,* free from nonprotein substances) but often occur as the protein portion of conjugated proteins, *e.g.,* globin from hemoglobin.

Globulins. Refers to class of proteins that are heat-coagulated and soluble in dilute solutions of salts; they differ from albumins in being insoluble in water. They are found in blood, *i.e.,* serum globins, in milk, *i.e.* lactoglobulins; and edestin from hemp seed and amandin from almond are also globulins.

Glucagon. An hormone which is secreted by the pancreas which causes an increased in blood sugar probably by increasing the breakdown of liver glycogen.

Glucaric Acid. Alternative name for saccharic acid, the dicarboxylic acid derived from glucose.

Glucide. Name occasionally used for saccharine.

Glucitol (glycitol). Obsolete names for sorbitol.

Glucoascorbic Acid. Homologue of ascorbinc acid having an extra CHOH group. Acts as an antagonist to the vitamin; its administration can cause scurvy in animals that do not normally need the vitamin in the diet.

Glucocorticoid. Obsolescent term for the steroid hormones of the adrenal cortex which affect carbohydrate metabolism.

Glucofuranose. Glucose which is formulated as the five-membered furan ring.

Gluconegenesis. Refers to the formation of glucose and glycogen from non-carbohydrate sources via glucose.

Gluconic Acid. Also termed dextronic acid, maltonic acid and glycogenic acid. It is formed by oxidation of the hydroxyl group on the first carbon of glucose.

Glucono-delta-lactone. Refers to lactone of gluconic acid. It slowly liberates acid at a controlled rate, and is used in chemically leavened bread, *i.e.,* to liberate carbon dioxide from bicarbonate instead of using yeast. Also used in bland-flavoured sherbets and to reduce fat-absorption in products like doughnuts.

Glucosaccharic Acid. Alternative name for saccharic acid.

Glucosamine. Amino derivative of glucose. Constituent of many complex polysaccharides.

Glucosan. A complex of glucose molecules, *e.g.*, starch, cellulose and glycogen. Insulin is a complex of fructose molecules and is a fructose molecules and is a fructosan.

Glucose. Also known as dextrose, grape sugar and blood sugar.

A simple six-carbon sugar (hexose) $C_6H_{12}O_6$, which is found naturally in plant tissue and formed by the hydrolysis of starch. It is the major product of the digestion of carbohydrates in the intestine and is the form in which the carbohydrate gets absorbed into the bloodstream. During digestion sucrose is hydrolysed to glucose and fructose, lactose to glucose and galactose, and starches and maltose to glucose.

Normal levels in blood lie between 80 and 100mg per

100ml, any surplus being converted to glycogen and stored as such in the liver and muscles. Glycogen is broken down to glucose when required for energy.

Energy gets liberated by the oxidation of glucose to carbon dioxide and water at the rate of 3.9 kcal per g or 686 kcal per gram-mol. It finds use in the manufacture of confectionery, since its mixture with fructose prevents sucrose from crystallising and it is less sweet than sucrose, being 74% as sweet.

Glucose Metabolism. Process through which glucose gets broken down in living tissues to provided energy. The overall reaction follows the equation.

$C_6H_{12}O_6 + 6O_2 \rightarrow 6CO_2 + 6H_2O$ + 3.9 kcal per gram of glucose but in detail the process involves about 20 stages.

Glucose Oxidase. Enzyme that specifically oxidises glucose to gluconic acid, with the formation of hydrogen peroxide.

Glucose Syrups. The term used for the purified, concentrated, aqueous solutions of nutritive saccharides from starch. Prepared by hydrolysis of maize starch (or potato starch) by enzymes, acid or a combination of the two. Usually 70% w/w total solids–glucose, maltose and oligomers of glucose of three, four or more units. These find used as a sweetening agent in sugar confectionery; also termed corn syrup, corn starch hydrous lysate, starch syrup, confectioners' glucose and uncrystallisable syrup.

Glucose Tolerance. Refers to the ability of the body to deal with a large dose of glucose, use as a test for diabetes mellitus.

The fasting subject ingests 50g of glucose and the blood sugar is measured at intervals. In the normal individual the fasting sugar level is approximately 80-100mg per 100ml, rises to about 150mg, and returns to the starting level with 1-1 1 over 2 hours. In diabetics the sugar rises to higher levels and takes longer to return. The plotted results form a glucose-tolerance curve.

Glucose-T_m. Term used in measuring the efficiency of the kidneys; it refers to the maximum rate of reabsorption of glucose by the kidney tubules. T_m is the maximum reabsorptive capacity.

Glucosides. Complexes of substances with glucose. General name for such complexes with other sugars is glycosides.

Glucostatic Mechanism. Refers to the theory that appetite depends on the difference decrease to 8mg% the hypothalamus gets stimulated and hunger results.

Glucuronic Acid. The acid which is derived from glucose by the oxidation of the group on C6. Many toxic substances get excreted from the body combined with glucuronic acid as glucuronides. It is also present in various complex polysaccharides.

Glutamic Acid. Refers to a dicarboxylic non-essential amino acid, amino-glutaric acid. Involved in transamination reactions, its amide is glutamine. The sodium salt, monosodium glutamate, MSG, originally called Aginomoto, is used to enhance flavour of savoury disches and is often added to caned meats and soups.

Glutamine. Amide of the amine acid glutamic acid which is formed by the addition of ammonia to glutamic acid. It is found in plants, where it appears to function as a storage depot for ammonia, and as part of the urea cycle in animals.

Glutathione. Refers to a tripeptide of glyucine; glutamic acid which is formed by the addition of ammonia to glutamic acid and cysteine. It occurs in animal tissues and believed to function as an oxidation-reduction system.

Glutelins. Refers to proteins which are insoluble in water and neural salt solutions but soluble ion dilute acids and alkalies, e.g., wheat glutenin.

Gluten. Refers to the protein complex in wheat, and to a lesser extent rye, which gives dough the viscid property that hold gas when it rise. None in oats, barley, maize. It has been a mixture of gliadin and glutelin.

In the undamaged state with extensible properties it is termed vital gluten, when overheated, these properties get lost and the product is called devitalised gluten.

Gluen-free Foods. Formulated without any wheat or rye protein (although the starch may be used) for subjects suffering from coeliac disease, which see.

Glutose. Ahexose sugar carrying a keto group on C_3. It is not metabolised and non-fermentable.

Glycamines. Derivatives of sugar alcohol in which the CH_2OH group is replaced by CH_2NH_2, e.g., ethanolamine and ribamine (part of vitamin B_2).

Glycerides. Esters of glycerol with fatty acids.

If all three molecules of fatty acid are the same, a simple triglyceride is formed, e.g., tristearin, triolein, mixed glycerides may be firmed such as distearo-olein and stearo-oleo-plamitin.

Glycerine. Glycerol.

Glycerol. A trihydric alcohol, chemically 1, 2, 3-propane troil, $CH_2OHCHOHCH_2OH$, popularly called glycine. Glycerol is a clear, colourless, odourless, viscous liquid, sweet to taste. Used as a solvent for flavours, as a humectant to keep foods moist, and in cake batters to improve texture and slow down staling.

Glycerose. Simple, three-carbon sugar, derived from the corresponding alcohol, glycerol. Formula. $CHOCHOHCH_2$ OH.

Glycerose Lactosterate. Also known as lactostearin which is formed by glycerolyses of hydrogenated soya bean oil followed by esterification with lactic acid, which result in a mixture of mono and diglycerides and their lactic mono esters. It finds use as an emulsifier in shortening.

Glycine. A non-essential amino acid, chemically amino acid, CH_2NH_2COOH. Chemically it finds use as buffer for gastric acidity.

It is having 70% of the sweetness of sucrose and is sometimes used mixed with saccharine as sweetening agent.

Glycionin. Globulli protein in soya bean.

Glycitols. Compounds with the general formula $CHOCCHOH_5CH_2OH$.; sugar alcohol, xylitol mannitol; also used previously as an alternative name for sorbitol itself.

Glycogen. Refers to storage form of carbohydrate in the animal body, in the liver and muscles. Composed of glucose units; is synthesised from the blood sugar and broken down to blood sugar as required. Sometimes referred to as animal starch.

Glycogeneses. Refers to the synthesis of glycogen from glucose, as, for example, occurs in the muscle where glucose is stored as glycogen; facilitated by insulin.

Glycogenolysis. Refers to breakdown of glycogen to glucose when this is required for the production of energy.

Glycolysis. There are two parts to the total breakdown of glucose. The first is anaerobic and called glucose fermentation of glycolysis. This ends at the formation of pyruvic acid. The second part is an oxidation and the series of reaction is the Krebs tricarboxylic acid cycle, or the citric acid cycle. This completes the breakdown to carbon dioxide and water.

Glycoproteins. Group of proteins which are conjugated with carbohydrates like uronic acids, polymerised glucosaminemannose, etc. including mucins and mucoids; found in the evitreous homour of the eye, cornea, cartilage, gastric mucosa.

Glycosides. Compound having a sugar attach to another molecule. When glucose is the sugar, they are termed as glucosides. A wide variety occur in plants and some are useful medicinally, such as digitalis and rutin.

Glycosuria. The term used for the appearance of glucose in the urine, as in diabetes and after the administration of drugs that lower the renal threshold.

Glycyrrhiza. Liquorice, Glycyrrhiza glabra. Extract of root long used to flavour medicines because of sweet taste due to calcium and potassium salts of glycyrhizic acid.

Glycyrrhizin. Triterpenoid glycoside which is extracted from liquorice root. It is 5–100 times as sweet as sucrose but with liquorice flavour. It is used to flavour tobacco and pharmaceutical substances, and as foaming agent in some non-alcoholic beverages.

GMS. Abbreviation for glyceryl monostearate.

Goitre. Enlargement of the thyroid gland which is seen as a swelling in the neck, due to deficiency of iodine in the diet and to the presence of 'goitrogens' in certain foods such as Brassicas and peanuts.

Supplementation with an iodide often disallows the condition, hence the use of iodised salts.

Goitrogens. Refers to the substances which are found in foods (especially of the Brassica species but including also groundnuts, cassava and soya bean) and interfere with normal functioning of the thyroid gland and can cause goitre in animals. They include glucosinolated (progoitrin), which prevent the synthesis of thyroxine in the thyroid gland, and thiocyanates, which interfere with the uptake of iodine. Progoitrin gets converted into active–5-vinyloxazolidine-2 thione. It is not clear that these substances are a cause of goitre in human beings.

Gold Thioglucose. Chemical which is used to causes obesity in experimental animals by stimulation of the appetite through damage to the hypothalamus.

Gooseberry. Berry of shrub, Ribes grossularia.

Analysis per 100g: protein 1g, fat 0.4g, kcal 42 (0.18MJ), Ca 22mg, Fe 0.5mg, carotene 90g, vitamin $B_1$0.04mg, vitamin B_2 0.02mg, nicotinic acid 1mg, vitamin C33mg.

Gooseberry, Cape. Edible fruit of Physalis Peruvians, also called golden berry.

Analysis per 100g : carbohydrate 9g, protein 2g, 48 kcal (200kJ), 600μg carotenen, approximately 30mg vitamin C.

Gooseberry, Indian. Emblic.

Gossypol. Yellow toxic pigment found up to 2–4% dry weight in some varieties of cottonseed (hexahydroxy) di-isopropyl dimethyl (binaphthalene) dicarboxyaldehyde. When included in chicken feed, it causes discoloration of the yolk. But has not been found to be toxic to man.

Gourds. Vegetable of the family Cucurbitaceae, including cucumber, marrow, pumpkin, squash, gourd and melon. All have more than 90% water and about 1% protein and have little food value apart from vitamin C at 10mg per 100g. In addition, yellow pumpkin contain 900μg carotene per 100g. Melons are sometimes grown for their seeds, which containd 20–40% oil and 20% protein.

Grahaum Bread. Whole-wheat bread in which the bran is very finely ground. Graham cakes are made from wholemeal flour and milk.

Gram-negative, Gram-positive. Bacteria can be divided into two groups, depending on whether or not they retain crystal-violet dye after staining and decolorising with alcohol. Named after Danish botanist Gram.

Grams, Indians. Name given to small dried peas, *e.g.* green gram (Phaseolus aureus), black gram (Phasecolus mungo), red gram (Cajanus indicus).

Grape. Fresh fruit of a large number of varieties of Vitis vinifera.

Can be grouped as dessert grapes, wine grapes and varieties that are used for drying to produce raisins, currants and sultanas. Contain only 3–4mg vitamin C per 100g.

Grapefruit. Fruit of Citrus paradise; thought to have arisen as a sport of pomelo or shaddock (Citrus grandis), a coarser citrus fruit, or as a hybrid between pomelo and sweet orane, 35–45mg vitamin C per 10g. The pity contain naringin, which is very bitter.

Grade Sugar. Alternative name for glucose.

GRAS. 'Generally regarded as safe'. Designation give to food additives when further evidence is required before the substance can be classified more precisely.

Grass Tetany. Magnesium deficiency in cattle.

Gratin. Gratin is French term for the thin brown crust formed on top of foods that have been covered with butter, breadcrums or cheese and heated under the grill or in the oven.

Au gratin is the term used when cheese is used.

Gratin is also the name given to a fireproof dish, and the verb is gratiner.

Gray (Gy). The SI unit for ionising radiation instead of the rad—the gray is equivalent to 1J/kg (=100 rad).

Green S. Food colour also known as Wool green S and Brilliant acid green BS; sodium salt of di-(*p*-dimethyl-aminophenyl)-2 hydroxy 3, 6-disulphonaphthyl-methanol anhydride.

Grill. To cook by radian heat; some of the fat is lost. Barbecues cook by grilling.

Grissinl. Italian 'Finger rolls' or stick bread 6–18 inches long.

Grist. Cereal for grinding.

Groats. Oats from which the husk has been entirely removed; when crushed, Embden goats result.

GTF. Glucose tolerance factor.

Guarana. Dried paste prepared from the seeds of the climbing shrub Paullinia cupana (South America); rich in caffeine; used in South America as a beverage similar to cocoa.

Guar Gum. Cyamopsis gum; from the cluster bean, Cyamposis tetragonoloba. Member of Leguminosae, used in India as livestock feed. The gum is a water-soluble, galactomannan; used 'slimming' preparations, as it is not digested by digestive enzymes, and in experimental treatment of diabetes, since it delays gastric emptying and prevents a rapid rise in blood sugar.

Guava. Fruit of Psidium guajava, tropical shrub (Central and South America), eaten raw or preserved as guava jelly.

Gum Arabic. Exudate from the stems of several species of acacia, also called gum acacia (best product comes from Acacia senegal). Used as thickening agent, as stabiliser often in combination with other gums, in gum groups and soft jelly gums and to prevent crystallisation in sugar confectionery.

Gum, Chewing. Based on chicle, the partially evaporated milky juice of latex of the Sapodilla tree, plus sugar, balsam of Tolu and flavour.

Gums. Refers to substances that can disperse in water on form a viscous, mucilaginous mass. Used in food processing to stabilise emulsions (such as salad dressings, processed cheese), as a thickener and in sugar confectionery. These are extracted from seeds (guar gum, locust, quince, psyllium), sap or exudates (gum arabic, karaya (or sterculia), tragacanth, ghatti, bassora or hog gum, shiraz, mesquite, anguo) and seaweeds (agar, kelp, alginate, Irish moss) or they may be made from starch or cellulose (dextrins and methyl-, carboxymethy1-, etc. cellulose) or they may be synthetic, such as vinyl polymers.

Most of these (apart from dextrins) are not digested and are having no food value.

Gum Tragacanth. It is obtained from the trees of Astralagus species: used as stabiliser.

H

Haematin. Formed by the oxidation of haem, the non-protein part of hemoglobin; the iron gets oxidised from the ferrous to the ferric state.

Haemin. Refers to the hydrochloride of haematin which is derived from hemoglobin. The crystals are readily recognisable under the microscope and used as a test for blood.

Hemoglobin. Refers to the red colouring matter of the red blood cell, which is composed of the protein globin, combined with an iron containing pigment, haem. Hemoglobin combines reversibly with oxygen, which it carries from the lungs, to the tissues, and with carbon dioxide, which it carries from the tissues to the lungs, where it is excreted. In iron-deficiency anemia there occurs a deficiency of hemoglobin and impaired oxygenation.

Haemoglobinometer. An instrument which is used to measure the amount of hemoglobin in blood by direct colorimetry or after conversion to another coloured compound.

Haemoglobinometer. An instrument which is used to measure the amount of hemoglobin in blood by direct colorimetry or after conversion to another coloured compound.

Haemosidrin. Storage form of iron formed when there is excess available.

Hagberg Test. Measure of alpha-amylase activity of flour which is derived from the change in viscosity flour paste.

Haggis. Traditional Scottish dish which is prepared from liver, heat and lungs of sheep, cooked with suet, oatmeal and seasoning, then filled into a bag made from sheep's stomach and boiled for several hours.

Half-life. In biochemistry it refers to the time taken for half of the body tissue in question to be replaced.

Halibut Liver Oil. One of the riches natural sources of vitamins A and D. It is having 5g vitamin A and 8mg vitamin D per 10g.

Halophilic Bacteria. Able to grow in high concentrations of salt (25%). Colon group of bacteria get inhibited at 8–9% salt, Clostridia at 7–10%, food poisoning stphylococci at 15-20%, Penicillium 20%; film-forming yeasts can grow in 24% brine.

Halva. Also spelled halawa, halawa and chalva. A sweetmeat which is composed of an aerated mixture of glucose, sugar and crushed sesame seeds; because of the sees, the sweet is having 25% fat.

Ham. The whole hind leg of the pig removed from the carcase and cured individually; sometimes the process is secret.

Hammarsten's Casein. A casein which is prepared by the method of Hammarstein. Fat-free milk diluted with water and precipitated with acetic acid. Washed three times with water by decantation; dissolved in ammonium hydroxide and reprecipitated, this repeated twice. The final precipitate washed with alcohol and ether and finally extracted with ether in a Soxhlet.

Hammer Mill. Mill in which material has been powdered in impact from a set of hammers; a continuous process.

Hansa Can. An all-aluminium can (developed in Germany) with easily opened ends.

Hardening of Oils. Hydrogenated oils.

Hashish. Indian Hemp.

Haslet. (harslet). Old English country dish which is made from pit's offal (heart, liver, lungs and sweetbread) cooked in small pieces with seasoning and flour.

Hasty Pudding. Prepared from flour, milk, butter and spices, which, since they were usually readily available, could be quickly made into the pudding from unexpected visitors. Made in the USA with maize (corn) flour instead of wheat flour.

Haybox Cooking. The food is cooked for only a short time, then kept in a well-lagged container, the haybox, where it remains hot for many hour and so cooking continues without further use of fuel. Also known as the fireless cooker.

Haze. Term in general use in brewing to indicate cloudiness of the beer. Chill haze appears at °C but there is no fundamental difference. Due to gums derived from the barley, leucoanthocyanins from the malt and hops, and glucose, pentoses and amino acids.

HDL. High-density lipoproteins.

Headcheese. Chopped, cooked edible parts of meat or meat product, also known as mock brawn.

Health Foods. Substances whose consumption has been advocated by various reform movements, including vegetable foods, whole grain cereals, food processed without chemical additives, foods grown on organic compost, 'magic' foods (honey, molasses, yogurt, etc.) and pills and potions.

Heat Sugar. Inositol.

Heat Exchanger. An equipment which is used for heating or cooling liquids rapidly by providing a large surface area and turbulence for the rapid and efficient transfer of heat. Used for continuous pasteurisation and also for the subsequent cooling.

Heat of Combustion. Energy which gets released by complete combustion, as, for example, in the bomb calorimeter. Values can be used to predict energy available physiologically only if an allowance is made for material not oxidised in the body.

Hedonic Scale. Term used in tasting panels where the judge indicated the extent of his like or dislike for the food.

Heifer. Young cow that has never had a calf.

Hemicelluloses. Complex carbohydrates which are composed of polyuronic acids combined with xylose, glucose, mannose and arabinose. Found together with cellulose and lignin in plant cell walls; most gums and mucilages belong to this group of compounds.

Hemoglobin. Haemoglobin.

Haemosiderin. Haemosiderin.

Heparin. A substance which it isolated from liver, lung, muscle, heart and blood which prevents blood coagulation by acting as an antiprothrombin and an antithrombin. In vivo disappears rapidly from the blood stream, but in vitro 10mg prevents the coagulation of 10 ml of blood.

Hepatoflavin. Name given to substance which is isolated from liver, shown later to be riboflavin.

Herbs. Not clearly distinguished from spices, except that they usually refer to the whole of the soft-streamed aromatic plant, while spices are only part of the plant.

Herring Family. Herring is Clupea harangues; young herrings are sild. Spart is Clupea sprattus; young as brislings. Pilchard is Clupea pilchardus; young are sardines. Kippers, bloaters and red herrings are salted and smoked herrings; bucklings are ho-smoked herrings. Gaffelbitar are preserved herring.

Hesperidin. At one time called vitamin P, because it affects the fragility of the capillary walls. Found in the pity of the unripe orange and other citrus fruits; chemically a complex of glucose and rhamnose with the flavonone hesperin.

Hess Test. A test which is used for capillary fragility in scurvy. A slight pressure is applied to the arm for 5 minutes and shower of petechiae appear on the skin below the area of application.

Hexamic Acid. A synthetic sweetening agent; trade name (Abbott Laboratories) for cyclohexy; sulphamic acid (the free acid of cyclamage); 27 time as sweet as sugar. Used in effervescent drinks.

Hexoestrol. Synthetic oestrogenic hormone. It does not occur naturally.

Hexosans. The general name for complex polysaccharides built up from simple units of hexose sugars.

Hexose. A six-carbon sugar such as glucose and fructose.

Hexose Monophosphate Shunt. Refers to an alternative pathway in the metabolism of glucose to the Embden–Meyerhof–Parans pathway.

The glucose-6-phosphate formed in the main route can get converted to phosphoglucoine acid, then to pentose phosphate and to sedoheptulose-7-phosphate. The latter then joins the main pathway.

As pentoses are formed, it is also referred to as the pentose cycle and the direct oxidative pathway.

Hexuronic Acid. The acid which is derived from a hexose sugar by the oxidation of the group on C_6. The hexuronic acid derived from glucose is clucuronic acid.

HFCS. High-fructose corn syrup.

HF Heating. High frequency heating.

Hiochic Acid. Growth factor which was isolated in 1956 in Japanese rich wine (sake) and later shown to the identical with mevalonic acid.

Hirudin. Blood anticoagulant which is found in the buccal glands of the leech. It functions by interfering with thrombin.

Histamine. Compound which is formed from decarboxylation of the amino acid histidine, and also found in been-chocolate, sauerkraut, and wines in small amounts.

Histidine. An amino acid which is essential to the growing rat but not to adult man. It is assume that it is essential to the growing child. Chemically, amino iminazole propionic acid.

Decarboxylation produces histamine.

Histohaematin. Or myohaematin, earlier name for cytochrome, which see.

Histones. Proteins soluble in water but insoluble in dilute ammonia; yield precipitates with solutions of other proteins; on hydrolysis yield large quantities of argrinine and lysine.

HMS. Hexose Monophosphate Shunt.

HMT. Hexamethylen tetramine.

Hogget. One-year-old sheep.

Hogshead. For beer or cider has 54 gallons; for wind contains 52-1/2 gallons.

Holoenzyme. An enzyme protein together with its coenzyme or prosthetic group.

Holosides. Name assigned to complexes of sugars (or osides) that yield only sugars on hydrolysis. As distinct from heterosides, which yield other substances as well as sugars on hydrolysis, *e.g.* tannins, anthocyanis, nucleosids.

Hominy. Prepared maize kernels, Lye hominy–pericarp and germ removed by soaking in caustic soda. Peralied hominy–degermed hulled maize. Corn grits are ground hominy.

Hymocysteine. Refers to the demethylated from of the amino acid methionine, $SHCH_2CH_2CHNH_2COOH$. Does not occur in foods and is not nutritional importance, but of great biochemical interest as an intermediate in cell reactions. The non-essential amino acid systine is made from the essential methionine via homocysteine.

Homogenisation. Emulsions usually is having a suspension of globules varying size. Homogenisation reduces these globules to a smaller and approximately equal size.

In homogenised milk the smaller globule absorb more of the milk protein, which is a stabiliser, and the cream does not rise to the top.

Homiotherms. Animals that are able to maintain constant body temperature irrespective of the surrounding temperature; also known as warm-blooded animals.

Honey. Syrup liquid which is manufactured by bees from the nectar of flowers (ESSENTIALLY SUCROSE). The flavour and colour depend on the flower from which the nectar was obtained and the composition also varies with the source.

Average composition: water 18% (12-26%), invert sugars, *i.e.,* glucose and fructose, 74% (59-75%), sucrose 1.9% (0.4%), ash 0.18% (0.1-0.8%), organic acid 0.1-0.4%.

If the ratio between fructose and glucose is high, there occurs a tendency for the honey to crystallise.

Honeydew Honey. During periods of prolonged drought bees may supplement their nectar supplies with honeydew, the sweet fluid excreted on leaves by leaf-sucking insects. The resultant honey is dark having an unpleasant taste.

Hop. Refers to a perennial climbing plant, Humulus lupulus. The female flowers contain bitter resins and essential oils used in brewing beer.

Hordein. A protein in barley; one of the prolamines.

Horcdenin. Alkaloid occurring in germinated barely, sorghum and millet which can cause hypertension and respiratory inhibition.

Horlick's Trade name (Harlick'Ltd.) for a preparation of malted milk, for consumption as a beverage when added to milk.

Analysis per 100g: protein 14.4g, fat 8.0g, carbohydrate 70.8g, Ca 272mg, Fe 1mg kcal 400 (1.7MJ).

Hormones. Chemical agents which are produce in the body, also known as endocrines. Thyroxine and tri-iodothyronine from the thyroid, adrenaline from the adrenaline, insulin from the pancreas and a variety of hormones from the pituitary gland. They secreted directly into the blood stream from these ductless glands and act as chemical messengers which stimulate other tissues.

Hormones, Sex. Male hormones, or androgens, include testosterone and androsterone; female hormones, or oestrogens, include oestradiol, oestrone and progeterone. Chemically, all are steroid in structure.

Horsemeat. Analysis per 100g : protein 15g, fat 3g, kcal 94 (0.4MJ), Ca 8mg, Fe 1.8mg, vitamin A nil, vitamin B_1 0.05mg, vitamin B_2 0.08mg, nicotinic acid 3.2mg, vitamin C nil.

Hortvet Freezing Test. Test for the adulteration of milk with water by measuring the depression of freezing point; normal range–0.53 to–0.55C.

Hot Breads. Americanese for waffles and pancakes.

Hot Sause. A tomato sauce having hot flavour due to cayenne.

HPLC. High performance liquid chromatography.

HTST. High performance liquid chromatography.

HTST. High-temperature-short time treatment. It may be defined as sterilisation by heat from times ranging from a few seconds to 6 minutes; usually applied to flow sterilisation, in which the process time is less than about 1 minutes.

Humectant. Refer to a substance that absorbs moisture and used to maintain the water content of materials like tobacco, glue, inks, baked products, soaps, textiles. For example, glucose syrup, invert sugar, honey dried whey, glycerol, sorbitol. They allow the addition of sugar without adding more water and so prevent the growth of moulds.

Humidity. Relative humidity.

Humulone. One of the two resins which are found in hops, the other being lupulone. Humulone is a mixture of humulone, cohumulone and adhumulone. The resins have been responsible for bitter flavour of the hops used in brewing.

Hursting Mill. Horizontal stone grinders which were once used for grain milling.

Husk, or Hull. In reference to cereal grain, this is the outer woody cellulose covering. In wheat it is loosely attached and removed during threshing; in rice it is firmly attached. It is high in fibre content and of limited used as animal feed.

Hyaluronic Acid. The mucopolysaccharide which, in animal tissues, binds water in the interstitial spaces, and holds the cells together and acts as a schock-absorber in the joints; also present in the vitreous homour of the eye.

Its viscosity gets reduced by the enzyme hyaluronidase, by which it is depolymerised.

Hyaluronidase. A group of carbohydrase enzymes that are able to depolymerise mucopolysaccharides such as hyaluronic acid. Found in bee-sting, bacteria, tests, leeches.

Also known as spreading factor, as the enzyme breaks down the hyaluronic acid under the skins and permits the spread of substances there. For this reason it is used clinically to aid the absorption of drugs administered subcutaneously or intramuscularly, and to permit the subcutaneous injections of relatively large volumes of solution as, for example, in glucose feeding by this route.

Hydrocooling. Vegetables are washed in colled water, then, while still wet, subjected to vacuum. The evaporation of the water chills the vegetables for transport. The term is also applied to vegetables washed in ice water without the vacuum treatment.

Hydrogenated Oils. Liquid oils can be hardened by hydrogenation. Treatment with hydrogen in the presence of a nickel catalyst brings about 'saturation' of the double bonds of the fatty acid chain a raise in melting point. Cottonseed, maize, sunflower and whale oils are usually hardened and used in margarine and cooking fats.

Hydrogen-ion Concentration. Measure of the acidity or alkalinity of a solution by the concentration of hydrogen ions present.

Hydrogen Peroxide. Anti-microbial agent. It can be used at 0.1% to preserve milk (Buddesied milk), but destroys vitamin C, methionine and tryptophan.

Hydrostatic Steriliser. Refers to continuous steriliser in which the process is carried out under sufficient depth of water to maintain the required pressure. It is used for continuous sterilisation of canned foods on a large scale.

Hydroxybenzoic Acid Easters. Methyl, ethyl, propyl and butyl esters of hydroxybenzoic acid and their sodium salts; used as anti-fungal agents and preservations. Also called paraben esters.

Hydroxycholecalciferols. Vitamin D.

Hydroxylysine. Amino acid occurring only in connective tissue proteins of animals; incorporated into the protein as proline and then hydroxylated in the delta position.

Hydroxyproline. Amino acid found only in connective tissue proteins of animals; incorporated into the protein as proline and then hydroxylated. Peptides of hydroxyproline are excreted in the murine and the output gets increased when collagen turnover is high, as in rapid growth or resorption of tissue.

Hydroxyproline Index. Urinary hydroxyproline excretion is reduced in children suffering protein-energy malnutrition. The index refers to the ratio between hydroxyproline and creatinine per kg body weight and is low in malnourished children.

5-hydroxytryptamine. Or serotonin; 3-(2-aminoethy;)-5-indolol. Formed form the amino acid tryptophan; found in blood, and in high concentrations in the plantain; brings about vasco-constriction and is a neurotransmitter.

Hygorscopic. Readily absorbing water, as when table salt becomes damp. Materials such as calcium chloride and silica gel absorb water so readily that they are used as drying agents.

Hyperchlorhydria. Excess of hydrochloric acid in the stomach, due, not to higher concentration in the gastric juice, but to greater volume of secretion.

Hyperlipidaemias. Common disorder of affluent communities, in which there occurs an increased level of the plasma lipids–phospholipids, triglycerides, free and esterified cholesterol and unesterified farry acid.

Hyperthyroidism. Overactivity of the thyroid gland bring about increased basal metabolic rate.

Hypertonic. A solution which is more concentrated than isotonic, which see.

Hypervitaminosis. Overdosage with vitamins. In most cases there occurs no ill-effect, but hypervitaminosis A and also D have ill effects; overdosage with nicotinic acid brings about flushing of the face and neck.

Hypokalaemia. Refers to a fall in the level of blood potassium. (Latin name kalium).

sHypophysectomy. Refers to surgical removal of the pituitary gland (the hypophysis).

Hypoproteinaemia. Total plasma protein level less than 5.5g per 10ml (normally 6.7–7.7).

Hypothermia. Low body temperature which occurs among elderly far more easily than in younger adults, often with fatal results. Also is used in connection with reduction of body temperature down to 28°C to allow surgery of heart and brain.

Hypothyroidism. The term used for the underactivity of the thyroid glandism; thyroid gland.

Hypotonic. A solution which is more dilute than isotonic.

I

Inanition. Exhaustion and wasting because of complete lace of or non-assimilation of food; a state of starvation.

Inborn Errors of Metabolism. Genetic disease.

Index of Nutritional Quality (INQ). Refers to an attempt to provide an overall figure for the nutrient content of food or a diet. It may be defined as the ratio between the percentage of the recommended daily amount of each nutrient and the percentage of the RDA (which) for energy.

Indian Corn. Maize.

Indian Hemp. Or hashish, Cannabis indica; active principle unknown, stimulated and deranges the mental processes.

Indian Rice Grass. Perennial, growing wild in the USA, Oryzopsis hymenoids; tolerant to drought.

Seeds resemble millet, small, round, dark in colour covered with white hairs. Used by North American Indians for flour; now used almost exclusively for forage.

Indican

1. Metabolic indican is 3-indoxylsuphuric acid which gets excreted in urine of mammals and occur in blood plasma; derived from tryptophan.

2. Plant indican is 3-beta-glucosido-indole (indoxyl-glucoside) occurring in plants of Indigofera and some other species.

Indigo Carmine. Blue food colour, disodium salt of

indigotin-5.5'-disulphonic acid. Indigotin is the colouring principle of natural indigo which is obtained from the indigo fern. Permitted food colour in most countries but its use gets limited by its low stability and solubility.

Induction Period. Frequently used in connection with fasts. It refers to the lag period during which the fat show stability to oxidation due to its content of antioxidants, natural or added, which get preferentially oxidised. After this induction period there occurs a sudden and large consumption of oxygen and the fat becomes rancid.

Inorganic. Denoting of mineral as distinct from animal and vegetable origin. Apart from carbonates and cyanides, inorganic chemicals are those that contain no carbon.

Inosite. Obsolete name for inositol.

Inositol. Refers to essential nutrient for micro-organism and many animals and so classed as a vitamin, although there occurs no evidence of its essentiality for man. Deficiency causes alopecia in mice and 'spectacle eye' (denudation around the eye) in rats.

Chemically it is hexahydrocyclohexane $(CHOH)_6$. It occurs widely in plant and animal tissues as an essential part of the structure and in combination in phosphatides. Its hexaphosphoric acid ester is phytic acid.

Instant Food. Refers to the dried foods that reconstitute rapidly when water is added, *e.g.*, tea, coffee, milk, soups, precooked cereal products, potatoes, etc. Product may be agglomerated after drying to control particle size and improve solubility.

'Instant puddings' have been formulated with pregelatinised starch and disperse rapidly in cold milk.

Insulin. An hormone that controls carbohydrate metabolism. It is secreted by the pancreas gland. Diabetes mellitus (which) is due to underproduction or overdestruction of insulin. The hormone is a protein and is digested if given by mouth, so must be administered by injection. Cannot be synthesised and is prepared from animal pancreas.

Interesterifiction. Fats are mixture of triglycerides with various fatty acids esterified to the glycerol. By dry heat at 45–95°C there occurs an exchange of the farry acids between the glycerol molecules–interesterification–with a consequent change in physical properties of the fat. For example, lard is not a good creaming fat until is has been so treated.

Intermediate Moisture Foods. Contain 15–40% moisture.

International Units. Used as a measure of the comparative potency of natural substances, such as vitamins, before they could be obtained in sufficiently pure form to measure by weight. An international unit (i.u.) may be arbitrarily defined in terms of a reproducible standard, *e.g.* 1 i.u. of vitamin A was originally 1 microgram of the purest then known preparation of carotene, later 0.6 microgram of beta-carotene.

Intestinal Juice. Also called success entericus. Digestive juice produced by the intestinal glands lining the small intestine. Having the enzymes 'erepsin' (aminopeptidase and dipeptidase), amylase, maltase lactase, sucrose, lipase, esterase, nucleases, nucleotidase, and the activator enterokinase (activates trypsinogen and chymotrypsinogen of the pancreatic juice to trypsin and chymotrypsin).

Intestine. Loosely this term is used to describe the whole of the gastrointestinal tract; more specifically that part after the stomach-comprising small intestine (duodenum, jejunum and ileum) and large intestine.

Intestine, Small. Refers to that part lying between the stomach and the large intestine, comprising duodenum, jejunum and lieum. The site of the greater part of digestion of food and absorption of the products. Only water gets absorbed in the large intestine.

Intolerance (to tools). Refers to any adverse reaction ranging from lactose intolerance, to inborn errors of metabolosm, to allergy.

Intravenous Nutrition. Slow infusion of solution of nutrients into veins by catheter.

Intrinsic factor. Pernicious anaemia.

Inulin. A ploysaccharide which is composed of fructose units. It is produced in the dahlia tube and Jerusalem artichoke as a storage carbohydrate. It is used as a test of renal function.

Inversion. Applied to sucrose. This term means its hydrolysis to glucose and fructose.

Invertase. Enzyme that splits sucrose into the invert sugars, glucose and fructose. Also known as sucrase or saccharase.

Invert Sugar. Mixture of glucose and fructose which is produced by hydrolysis of sucrose, 130% sweetness of sucrose. Important in the manufacture of sugar confectionery sine the presence of 10–15% of invert sugar prevents the crystallisation of came sugar.

Iodine. A trace element which is required at the level of 150 micrograms per day. It is part of the hormone thyroxine produced by the thyroid gland, and a prolonged shortage of iodide in the diet leads to goitere.

Iodine Number. Iodine value.

Iodine Solution, Hubl's. Solution of iodine and mecuric chloride which is used to determine the iodine number of unsaturated compounds.

Iodine Value. Or iodine number. It refers to the measure of the degree of unstauration of a fat by the extent of the uptake of iodine (grams iodine per 10g of fat) by the unsaturated double bonds in the fatty acid chain.

Iodised Salt. Usually 1 part of iodide in 25000–50000 parts of salt.

Iodophors. Acidic solution os iodine complexed with non-ionic surface-active agent which release iodined when diluted with water and actas effective antibacterial agents at relatively low temperatures.

Ion-exchange Resins. Various resins, like Permutit, Zeocarb, Amberlite, Dowex, will absorb ions under one set of conditions and release them under other conditions. The best-known example has been in water softening, where the calcium ions are removed from the hard water by the resin, and liberated from the resin by the addition of salt (regeneration).

The ion-exchange resins have been used for purification of chemicals, metal recovery and analysis.

IQB. Individual quick blanch. It is a method of blanching food by subjecting each particle to steam for a relatively short time and then accumulating the food in a deep until equilibration of temperature occurs.

Irish Moss. Red seaweed, Chrondrus crispus. It is source of the polysaccharide carageenan.

Iron. A mineral essential to the body; the average adult is having 4–5g of iron, of which 60–70% is present as heam in the circulating hemoglobin, and the remainder present in various enzymes (*e.g.* catalase, cytochrome oxidase), in muscle myoglobin or stored.

Prolonged deficiency gives rise to nutritional anaemia.

Iron Ammonium Citrate. Ferric ammonium citrate.

Iron Caseinate. The term used for the preparation of iron and casein; also known as iron nucleo-albuminate.

Iron, Reduced. Metallic iron in finely divided from which is produced by reduction of iron oxide. The form in which iron is sometimes added to foods, such as bread.

Iron Vitellinate. The term used for the preparation of egg yolk and iron.

Irradiation. With reference to foods, three main types of irradiation are used: ultraviolet, ionising and high-frequency (or microwave). Ultraviolet irradiation (2100–2900 nm) is used to sterilise the surface of foods, and convert ergosterol and 7-dehydrocholesterol to ergocalciferol (vitamin D_2) and choleacalciferol (vitamin D_3), respectively.

Ionising irradiation from radioactive isotopes or the linear accelerator destroys micro-organisms and insects, and also inhibits sprouting of potatoes. If finds use at various levels of treatment.

(a) Redurisation refers to low doses adequate for reducting the numbers of spoilage organisms.

(b) Radicidation refers to doses sufficient to reduce the

number of specified viable non-sporing pathogens below detectable levels.

(c) Radappretisation is treatment with doses sufficiently great for reducing the numbers of organisms below detectable levels (so called commercial sterility).

(d) Radiopasteurisation sufficient to destroy most pathogens.

Microwave heating uses high-energy electromagnetic radiation (commonly 2350 MH_z, wavelength 12cm) which generates heat throughout the food. It finds use for domestic cooking, to reheat food in catering and to 'finish drying' some commercially manufactured foods.

Ishaemic Heart Disease. Or coronary heart disease. Group of syndromes which are arising from failure of coronary arteries to supply sufficient blood to heart muscles; associated with atherosclerosis of coronary arteries.

Isinglass. Protein membrane from the swim bladder of certain species of sturgeon; practically pure collagen. When specially prepared, is used to clarify beer as to slowly precipitates and carries with it any suspended particles.

Islets of Langerhans. Areas of the pancreas from which the insulin gets secreted.

Isoascorbic Acid. Erythorbic acid.

Isodesmosine. A complex cross-linked compound which is involving four lysyl residures formed, together with desmosine, in connective tissue.

Isoelectric Point. Proteins and amino acids carry both negative and positive charges on the molecule, and are therefore called amphoteric. At a certain degree of acidity, depending on the particular protein or amino acid, the substance gets electrically neutral, *i.e.* the isoelectric point.

Proteins are usually least soluble and therefore get precipitated from solution at the IEP.

Isoenzymes. Refers to a mixture of several different enzymes having similar biological activity. For example, tissue lactice acid dehydrogenase contains at least five components.

Isolencine. An essential amino acid which is rely limiting in foods-chemically, aminomethyl valeic acid.

Isomaltose. Also termed brachyose. Differs from maltose in that the two glucose units are linked 1,6 instead of 1,4. Unlike maltose, isomaltose is not fermented by yeasts; it is a reducing sugar.

Isomerase. Name given to the enzyme which is used to convert glucose into fructose, although its primary specificity is conversion of D-xylose to D-xylulose.

Isomers. Molecules containing the same atoms but differently arranged. They can be quite different compounds or closely related, as citric and isocitric acids, leucine and isoleucine.

Iso-osomotic. Isotonic.

Isoriboflavin. Refers to an analogue of riboflavin having the two methyl groups in the 5, 6 instead of the 6.7 position. It competes with the vitamin and so inhibits growth.

Isotonic. Two solutions are iso-osmotic (isosmotic) when they have the same total osmotic pressure. They are isotonic, relative to a particular semi-permeable membrane, when their effective osmotic pressures are the same, *i.e.* the osmotic pressure of their non-permeating ions.

If two isotonic solutions are separated by a semi-permeable membrane, there occurs not net movement of water across the membrane. For example, human blood plasma is isosmotic with 0.955% sodium chloride, and isotonic with 0.935% sodium chloride, since part of the osmoic pressure of the blood is due to its proteins, which are non-permeating.

Isotopes. Elements having the same chemical properties but differing only in their atomic weight.

Isotopes incorporated into physiological substances, like amino acids, enable those substances to get traced in their reactions in the body.

I.U. International unit.

J

Jamaica Ginger Paralysis. Refers to polyneurities which is caused by poisoning from an illicit extract of Jamaica ginger ('jake) affecting thousands of people in the USA in 1930. Due to triorthocresyl phosphate.

Jamaica Pepper. All pice.

Jejunum. Refers to the second portion of the small intestine between the duodenum and the ileum.

Jelly. Refers to a colloidal suspension that has set; may be made from gelatin, pectin, agar, usually flavoured with fruit juice or synthetic flavour.

Jerked Beef. Dried meat of South America, similar to biltong.

Jesuit's Bark. Cinchona bark, source of quinine.

Jonathan. Refers to calcined, ground oat chaff used as adulterant for maize and other cereals (mid-nineteenth century).

Judas Goat. Sheep cannot readily be driven to slaughter but will follows a goat. A Judas goat is used to lead the sheep to the killing pens.

Julienne. Vegetables which are cut into thin, match-like strips. Also a clear, vegetables soup.

Junket. Refers to the precipitated protein of milk (casein only) which is carrying fat with it and leaving behind the clear whey. The precipitation is carried out with the enzyme rennin.

K

Kebab. General name (Oriental) for meat, usually two or three kinds, grilled on charoal; the pieces of meat are interpersed with vegetables.

Kebobs. An Indian dish: slices of mutton or fowl dipped in eggs and cooked on skewer.

Kedgere. An Indian dish of rice, split pulse, onions, eggs etc.; European dish of fish, rice eggs, etc. (Hindustani, khichri).

Kelp. Refers to any of several species of genus Laminaria– large brown seaweeds. Occasionally it finds use as food or food in gradient but mostly the ash is used as a source of alkali and iodine. Sometimes climbed a 'health' food with unspecified properties.

Kempner Diet. Or rice diet. A diet low in salt, comprising rice, fruit, fruit juices, sugar and vitamins, having about 2000 kcal (8. 4MJ), 15-30g protein and 100-150mg sodium per day, for patient suffering from congestive heart failure, cirrhosis of the liver, hypertensive disease, toxemias of pregnancy and certain kidney disorders.

Keyhalins. Or cephalins; phosphatides similar to lectins but composed of glycerol, fatty acids, phòsphoric acid and ethanolamine (instead of choline). These occur in brain and nerve tissue; part of cell structure.

Keratin. Insoluble protein of hair, horns, hoofs, feather and nails.

Ketchup (catsup or catchup). From the Chinese koechap or kitsiap, originally meaning brine of pickled fish. Now it is used for a spicy sauce or condiment made with juice of fruit or vegetable, vinegar and spices. Tomato ketchup has been a common sauce.

Ketogenic Diet. A diet which is poor in carbohydrate 920-30g but rich in fat; causes accumulation of the ketone bodies in the tissues used to be used in the treatment of epilepsy.

Ketonaemia. Refers to the accumulation in the blood of ketone bodies.

Ketone Bodies. Name assigned to the penultimate products of fatty acid metabolism–acetoacetic acid, betahydroxybutyric acid and acetone. They can get oxidised at only a limited rate, and when their production rate is excessive, as in diabetes and starvation, they accumulate in the blood (ketonaemia), and get excreted in the urine (ketonuria).

Ketonic Rancidity. Certain moulds of Penicillium and Aspergillus species attack fats having short carbon chains and produce ketones having a characteristic odour and taste–to-called ketonic rancidity. Fats like butter, coconut and palm kernel are most susceptible.

Ke tonuria. Ketone bodies.

Ketosis. Refers to clinical condition in which ketone bodies accumulate in the blood and appear in the urine.

Khushkhash. Israeli term for the bitter orange.

Kidney Clearance Test. Test of kidney function by measuring the ability to excreted per minute divided by the amount present in 1m/ of plasma gives the urinary clearance.

Kilocalorie. Calorie.

Kinetic Energy. Energy.

Kipper. Herring that has been lightly salted and smoked.

Kitol. Refers an inactive form of vitamin. A which is found in whale liver kitos, Greek for whale. It is converted into retinol by heating at 200°C.

Kjeldhal Determination. A method of determining total

nitrogen in a substance by digesting with sulphuric acid and a catalyst in a Kjeldahl (long-necked) flask. The nitrogen gets converted to ammonia which is then measured.

In foodstuffs most of the nitrogen is protein, and the term crude protein is the total 'Kjeldahl nitrogen' multiplied by the factor 6.25.

Klipfish. Salted and dried cod, mainly produced in Norway. The fish is boned, stored in salt for a month, washed and dried slowly. It is termed as bacalao in South America.

Kofranyi-michaelis Spirometer. An instrument that records the volume of expired air and takes samples at intervals for subsequent analysis. It thus serves as an indirect measure of the energy expended by the subject (indirect calorimetry).

Koji. Refers to a fungal proteolytic enzyme preparation from the mould. Aspergillus oryzae traditionally grown on steamed rice. Used to prepare products like miso by the proteolysis of soya, and soya sauces.

Kosher. Refers to the selection and preparation of foods in accordance with traditional Jewish ritual and dietary laws.

The only kosher flesh foods are from animals that chew the cud and have cloven hoofs, such as cattle, sheep, goats and deer, and the hindquarters must not be eaten. The only fish permitted are those with fins and scales, birds of prey and scavengers are not kosher. Moreover, the animals must not be eaten. The only fish permitted are those with fins and scales, birds of prey and scavengers are not kosher. Moreover, the animals must be slaughtered according to ritual before the mean can be regarded kosher.

Kerbs'Solution. Refers to the solution of inorganic salts with ionic composition similar to that of mammalian blood serum, with the addition of glucose, tissue slices contained to respire in such a solution. (Contains Na, Ca, Mg, K, Cl, PO_4, SO_4, HCO_3, CO_2).

Kries Test. For oxidative rancidity of fat. Fat treated with a solution of phloroglucinol in ether and hydrochloric acid–a pink colour develops in rancid fat, because of the presence of epihydrin aldehyde.

Krill. Term that refers to many specied of planktonic crustaceans but is mostly used in connection with the shrimp Euphausia superba. This is the main food of whales, certain types penguins and seabirds, occurs in shoals in the Antarctic, containing up to $12kg/m^3$. Contains 15% protein and is collected in limited quantities for use as human food.

Kryptoxanthin. Alternative spelling of cryptoxanthin, which see.

Kumquat. A citrus fruit of the genus Fortunella, widely distributed in S. China, resembles citrus fruits, but very small, acid pulp, and sweet, edible skin.

Kunitz inhibitors. Refers to protease inhibitors found in soyabeans together with another type called the Bowman–Brik inhibitors.

Kurrat. Plant closely related to leek.

L

Laccase. An enzyme in bacteria, potato and mushrooms that converts polyphenols to quinines.

Lacquer. In reference to tinned foods, this term refers to a layer of gum and gum coated onto the tinplate and hardened with heat. The layer of lacquer protects the tin lining from attack by acid fruit juices.

Lactalbumin. Refers to one of the proteins of milk casein 3%, lactalbumin 0.5%, lactogobulin 0.25%. Not precipitated from acid solution as casein is, hence, during cheese-making the whey is having the lactabumin and lactoglobulin. They are precipitated by heat, and a whey cheese can be made in this way.

Lactase. An enzyme that splits milk sugar, lactose, into glucose and galactose. It is present in the pancreatic juice.

Lactein Bread. Refers to another name for milk loaf, *i.e.*, loaf to which skim milk power has been added.

Lactic Acid. The acid which is produced by the fermentation of milk sugar and responsible for the flavour of sour milk and precipitation of the casein curd in cottage cheese. It is also produced by fermentation in silage, pickles, sauerkraut, cocoa, tobacco–its values here is in suppressing the growth of unwanted organisms. If finds use as an acidulant (as well as citric and tartaric acids) in sugar confectionery, soft drinks, pickles and sauces.

Lactobiose. Lactose.

Lactochrome. Pigment in milk.

Lactoflavin. Obsolete name for vitamin B_2; so named because it was isolated from milk.

Lactollin. Protein found (1962) in small traces in bovine milk, of unusual composition which is lacking methionine and with little alanine.

Lactometer. A floating device which is used to measure the specific gravity of milk (1.027-1.035).

Lac-tone. A protein-rich baby food (26% protein) which is made in Indian from peanut flour, skim milk power, wheat flour and barley flour with added vitamins and calcium.

Lacto-ovo-vegetarian. Refers to one whose diet is composed of vegetables, fruit, milk and eggs but no flesh foods.

Lactose. Milk sugar, 4.8% of milk. A disaccharide that gets hydrolysed by acid or the enzyme lactase to glucose and galactose. Fermented by micro organisms to lattice acid, hence the souring of milk by lactobacilli. It finds use pharmaceutically as tablet filler and as medium for growth of micro-organisms.

Ordinary lactose is alpha lactose (16% of the sweetness of sucrose), if crystallized above 93C, is changed to the beta form, which is more soluble and sweeter than the alpha form.

Lactulose. A synthetic disaccharide, galactosidofructose, which does not occur in nature. It is not digested, and when it is added in small amounts to infant milk formulas, the bacteria in the colon ferment it to lactic acid, so lowering the pH of the faeces in a way similar to that of human milk.

In larger amounts it acts as laxative, half as sweet as sucrose.

Laeotrile. Name given to extract of apricot kernels–amygdalin (a glucoside of benzaldehyde and cyanide). Claimed as a cure for cancer.

Lamb. Meat from sheep younger than 12-14 months.

Genuine spring lamb, 3-6 months; spring lamp up to 1 year.

Lanoline. The fat from wool. Consists of mixture of cholesterol oleate, cholesterol palmitate and cholesterol stearate, and used in various cosmetics.

Larch Gum. Refers to polymer of 1 part arabinose and 6 parts galactose found in the aqueous extract of the Western larch tree (Larix occidentals); potential substitute for gum arabic, because it is readily dispersed in water.

Lard. Best quality from fat surrounding stomach and kidneys of pit, but also from sheep and cattle.

Lard Compounds. Blends of animal fats, such as oleosterain or premier jus, with vegetable oils to produce products similar to lard in consistency and texture. Vegetable shortenings made from mixtures of partially hardened vegetable fats with the consistency of lard are referred to as lard substitutes.

Larding. Method of adding fat to learn meat so that it does not dry during long slow cooking. Narrow strips of bacon fat, 1-11/2 inches long and 3/4 inch wide, are threaded into the surface of the meat with a special larding needle. The strips are termed as lardoons. Barding is the process of tying a thin sheet of bacon fat over the meat.

Lard, Leaf. Made from the residue of kidney and back fat after the preparation of neutral lard at (50C) by treating with water above 100C in an autoclave.

Lard, Neutral. Highest-quality pig fat, which is prepared by agitating the minced fat with water at a temperature below 50C. Kidney fat provides No.1 quality; back fat provides No.2 quality.

Lthyrism. Refers to spastic paralysis of the lower limbs caused by high intake of Lathyrus sativus (Kesari dhal), which contain the neurotoxin β–N–oxalyl-amino-1-alanine (BOAA).

Lauric Acid. A long-chain fatty acid, $CH_3(CH_2)_{10}COOH$ occurs as the triglyceride in seeds of the spice bush and to lesser extent in butter, coconut oil and palm oil.

Laver. Edible seaweed. Laver bread is made from the seaweed Porphyra by boiling in salted water and mincing to a gelatinous mass. It is prepared into a cake with oatmeal or fried.

Laxative. Refers to a substance that accelerates the passage of food through the intestine. If it alters peristalitic activity, it is termed a purgative; other types stimulate or depress the muscular activity of the gut. Cellulose acts as a spurgative by retaining water and increasing the volume of instestinal contents; Epsom salts function similarly through osmotic pressure. Castor oil gets hydrolysed by lipase to liberate ricinoleic acid which irritates that intestinal mucosa. Drugs such as aloes, senna, cascara, rhubarb, and phenolphthalein irritate the intestine.

Lean Body Mass. Refers to the measure of body composition excluding adipose tissue, *i.e.,* cells, extracellular fluid and skeleton.

Leaven. Yeast. It is also used for a mixture of yeast, sugar and a small amount of flour which has already started to ferment and so is ready to add to the flour dough to make a loaf.

Lecithins. Refers to fatty substances of the type called phosphatides; consist of glycerol, fatty acids, phosphoric acid and choline. Important in the body for fat transport. It finds use in food technology as emulsifiers, *i.e.* in chocolate; help emulsification; save cocoa butter, and prevent bloom. Also used as anti-spattering agents in frying fats. Obtained commercially from soyabean, peanut and corn.

Lectins. Refers to toxic substances found in many legumes which cause red blood cells to agglutinate in vitro. Raw or undercooked beans of some varieties of Phaseoluls vulgaris cause vomiting and diarrhoea within 2 hours of consumption due to the high level of lectins but they are rapidly destroyed by boiling.

Leek. Allium ampeloprasum. It is a member of the onion family which has been known as a food for over 4000 years (eaten by the Israelites at the time of the Exodus from Egypt). The lower part is generally balanced by planting in trenches or earthling up, and is eaten along with the upper long green leaves.

Legumes. Refers to the seeds of the Leguminosae, including peas, beans and pulses. There is no difference between the terms 'peas' and 'beans' apart from common usage; the term 'pulses' or 'grain legumes' refers to the dried seeds; as distinct from the immature seeds eaten with the pod, oilseeds, soya beans and groundnuts (although the last two are members of the Leguminosae).

Legumin. Globulin protein in pea, bean and lentil.

Hehmann Process. Refers to a method of treating straw to render it digestible by cattle. The straw gets chopped and soaked in 1.5% sodium hydroxide, when it is delignified. The process raises the starch equivalent by a factor of 3–4.

Lemon. Fruit of Citrus lemon; having 40-60mg vitamin C per 100g fruit or pea 100ml juice.

Lemon Curd. Cooked mixture of sugar, butter eggs and lemons.

Lemons Oil. Refers to the peel oil-0.15–0.3% of the weight of the fruit; 90% limonene, together with phellandrene, terpinene, camphene, bisabolene, cadinene, citral, etc.

Lenhartz Diet. For peptic ulcer patients mainly fluid dies including raw eggs, milk, boiled rich and vegetable purees fed at frequent intervals.

Lentils. Seeds of many varieties of Lens esculenta. They fall into the same group as peas and beans. There is a green variety and an organce-red variety. Frequently used as a soup thickener in the power form.

Lettuce. Leaves of the plant Lactuca satins. It is not a very valuable food; the vitamin C is only one-seventh of that of cabbage.

Leucine. Refers to an essential amino acid; rarely limiting in foods. Chemically, amino isocaproic acid.

Leucocytes. White blood cells, normally 5000–9000 per cubic milimetre; include polymorphonuclear neutrophils, lymphocytes, monocytes, polymorphonuclear eosinophils, and polymorphonuclear basophils. A 'white cell count' determines the total; a 'differential cell count' estimates the number of each type.

Fever, haemorrhage, violent exercise cause an increase–leucocytosis; starvation and debitating conditions cause a decrease–leucopoenia.

Leucocytosis. Refers to increase in the white cells in the blood.

Leucopoenia. Refers to decrease in the white cells in the blood.

Leucosin. One of the water-soluble protein of wheat flour.

Leucovorin. Growth factor for Leuconostoc citrovorum. It is related to folic acid.

Levans. Polymers of fructose (principal one is inulin) which occur in tubers and some grasses; hydrolysed to fructose.

Levitin. Refers to one of the proteins of egg yolk, about one-fifth of the total, the remainder being vitellin. Rich in sulphur and accounts for half of the sulphur in the yolk.

Libermann-Burchard Reaction. Refers to the test for unsaturated sterols; green colour when treated with chloroform, acetic anhydride and concentrated sulphuric acid.

Lights. Butchers' term for the lungs of an animal.

Ligin. Associated with the carbohydrates of the cell wall of plants but not, itself, a carbohydrate, but a high molecular weight aromatic compound.

Legnoceric Acid. Long-chain fatty acid having total of 24 carbon atoms (tetracosanoic acid); present in the cerebrosides and sphingomyelins.

Lime. Fruit of Citrus aurantifolia which is cultivated almost solely in the tropics, since it is not as hard grow as other citrus fruits. Used to prevent scurvy. Contain about 10–20mg vitamin C per 100g fruit of fresh juice.

Limit Dextrin. When a branched polysaccharide like glycogen is hydrolysed enzymically (*e.g.* by phosphorylase), glucose is split of step by step until the branch point is reached. The hydrolysis then stops, leaving what is termed a limit dextrin. Further hydrolysis needs a different enzyme.

Limonin. Biter principle in the albedo of the Valencia orange.

Linamarin. Cyanogenetic glucoside which occurs in cassava (maniac) which may be a cause of neuropathies is are where cassava is a major food. Usually the cyanide is removed by enzymic action initiated by grating the tuber and then exposing to the air.

Linoleic Acid. Straight-chain fatty acid with 18 carbon atoms and two double bonds (a diene): $C_{17}Hs_{31}COOH$, with double bonds at 9–10 and 12–13 carbons (octadecadienoic acid).

Linolenic Acid. Refers to a straight-chain fatty acid of 18 carbon atoms with three double bonds: $C_{17}H_{29}COOH$, with double bonds at 9–10, 12–13 and 15–16 carbons (octadecatrienoic acid). It is a major component of linseed oil and its high degree of unsaturation has been responsible for the drying properties of the oil. At one time it was included with the essential fatty acids.

Lintner Value. Refers to a measure of diastatic activity using soluble starch as a substrate and measuring the effect by Fehling's solution. Applied to flour, malt extract, etc.

Liothyronine. Alternative name for L-tri-iodo thyronine, the most potent of the hormones of the thyroid gland. Used as an aid to weight reduction by stimulating the metabolism of the body.

Lipase. An enzyme that hydrolyses fat to glycerol and fatty acid. Having a low specificity and will attack any triglyceride or longchain ester. Present in the intestional juice and in many seeds and grains. Sometimes it is responsible for development for rancidity in stored foods.

Lipids (lipids, lipins). General term which is embracing fats, oils, waxes, complex compounds such as phosphatides and cerebrosides, sterol esters and terpenes. Their common property is insolubility in water and solubility in non-polar solvents, including chloroform, hydrocarbons and alcohols. Most include fatty acids in their structure.

Lipids, Plasma. Triglycerides, free and esterified cholesterol and phospholipids found in the blood plasma bound in specific lipoprotein complexes.

Lipocaic. Refers to unidentified factor in the pancreas that prevents the deposition of fat in the liver.

Lipochromes. Plant pigments which are soluble in fats and organic solvents, *e.g.* chlorophyll, carotenoids.

Lipofuscin. Group of pigments that accumulate in several body tissues, particularly the myocardium, during life and are consequently associated with the aging process.

Lipoic Acid. Essential growth factor for various micro-organisms.

In combination with vitamin B_1, phosphate and coenzymen A, lipoic acid forms lipothiamide, essential for the oxidative decarboxyliation in carbohydrate metabolism.

Lipolysis. The splitting of fats (to glycerol and fatty acid).

Lipolytic. Fat-splitting. Lipases are lipolytic enzymes.

Lipolytic Rancidity. Some micro-organisms give rise to lipases, and these fat-splitting enzymes are also present in tissue. In stored foods they hydrolyse the fats to free fatty acids–so called lipolytic rancidity. As the enzyme gets destroyed by heat, this type of rancidity occurs only in uncooked foods.

Lipovitellenin. Refers to a lipoprotein complex of egg comprising about one-sixth of the solids of the yolk.

Liqueurs. Distilled, flavoured and sweetened liquors from fermented sugar. For example, curacao 30% (w/v alcohol), 30% sugar, cherry brandy 19% alcohol, 33% sugar? advocate 14% alcohol 30% sugar, 0.75% nitrogen.

Liquefied Herring. Herring reduced to liquid state by enzyme action at slightly acid pH. It is used a protein concentrate for animal feed.

Litchi. Litchi chinenis, also lychee; native of China; the size of a small plum, with a translucent white jelly-like

Malting. Beer.

Maltitol. Refers to a polyol sweetner, 400-α-D-gluclpyranosyl-D-sorbitol, which is produced by hydrogenation of maltose. Hydrolysed in the lysed in the digestive tract to glucose and sorbitol and fairly completely utilised, providing 4 kcal per gram.

Maltol. Also called laxaarinic acid, palatone, veltol;3-hydroxy-2-methy-γ-pyrone. Found in the bark of young larch trees, pine needless, chicory and roasted malt; synthesised for use as a fragrant, caramel-like flavour for addition to foods. It imparts a 'freshly backed' flavour to bread and cakes.

Maltose. Malt sugar, maltobiose; 4-O-α-D-glucopyranosyl-D-glucopyranose. Double molecule of glucose which gets hydrolysed during digestion to glucose.

Manganese. Constituent of at least three mammalian enzymes and therefore a dietary essential, although dietary deficiencies have not been reported. Toxicity has been found among manganese miners. Deficiency in animals gives rise to defects in the synthesis of mucopolysaccharides.

Mangelwuzel, Mangoldwutzel. Beta vulgaris rapa. Cross between red and white beetroot, used as cattle food.

Mango. Mangifera indica. Fruit of Indo-Burmese origin which it extensively grown throughout the tropics; 3–6 inches diameter; organce-coloured edible flesh surrounding central stone. The depth of colour is an index of vitamin A activity, which can be up to 700μg per 10g.

Mangosteen. Fruit of Indian origin. The size of an orange with thick purple rind and sweet white pulp in segments (Garcinea mangostana). Vitamin C content 9mg per 100g.

Manna. Refers to the dried exudate from the manna-ash tamarisk tree (Fraxinus ornus). Abundant in Sicily and used as a mild laxative for children.

Mannitol. Mannite, or manna sugar. Formed by hydrogenation of the hexose sugar mannose. Also extracted commercially from seaweed (Laminaria).

Mannose. Also termed seminose and carubinose. Hexose sugar occurring in small amounts as polysaccharide complexes (mannosans) in legumes, in manna (exudate of the tamarisk) and in some gums.

Maple Syrup. Sap of certain varieties of the maple tree. Acer saccharum (USA and Canada). Evaporated either to syrup or finally to sugar. Malpe syrup, 62.6% sucrose, 1.5% invert sugar.

Maple Syrup Urine Disease. Refers to an inborn error or metabolism in which unusually large amounts of the three amino acid leucine, isoleucine and valine get exerted in the urine; the urine smells like maple syrup. There is progressive cerebrodegenearation leading to early death.

Marinade. A preparation of wine or vinegar with olive oil, lemon juice and herbs and spices. It used to soak meat or fish both to five flavour and to tenderise. Anchovy and Bismarck herrings are marinated before cooking.

Marjoram. Dried leaves of a number of aromatic plants of different species; Origanum majorana (perennial bush) and a sweet marjoram majorana hortensis (annual) maštichina. The volatile oils contain terpenes and terpene alcohols. Used as seasoning for poultry and meats.

Marmalade. Originally a jam which is made from the Portuguese marmelo or quince. Now the name given to jam made from citrus fruits such as orange, line, lemon, grapefruit.

Marmite.

1. The original form of pressure cooker which was used by Papin in 1681; it was an iron pot with a sealing lid.
2. Cookery term for a stock.

Marshmallow. Soft sweetmeat which is made from an aerated mixture of gelatin or egg albumin with sugar or starch syrup. Differs from nougat in containing less glucose and more water.

Marzipan. Sweetmeat or cake decoration which is composed of 25% ground almond past and 75% sugar; also called almond paste.

Marshing. In the brewing of beer, the malted barely is heated with water both to extract the soluble sugars and to continue enzymic reactions started during malting.

Mash Tun. A vessel which is used in brewing in which the malt is extracted from the sprouted barley with hot water.

Masecuite. The mixture of sugar crystals and syrup mother liquor which is obtained during the crystallisation stage of sugar refining.

Matoke. Cooked (steamed) green banana.

Maturation Factor. Refers to the substance in the liver which aids maturation of red blood cells. May be vitamin B_{12} or combination of B_{12} with the intrinsic factor produced by the stomach.

Matzka Process. Refers to the sterilisation by combined used of silver ions (oligodynamic process) and limited heat–katadyn process employes silver ions alone. In the presence of the silver the pasteurisation temperature is only 8–11C (15–20F). Applied to fruit juices.

Matzo, Motza. (matzoh is the plural). The term used for the unleavened bread or Passover bread made as thin, flat, round or square water biscuits, and, according to the injunction in Exodus, eaten by Jews during the eight days of Passover in place of leavened bread.

Maw. Fourth stomach of the ruminant.

Mawseed. Poppyseed.

Maysin. Coagulabe globulin protein of maize.

Meat. Generally this term refers to the muscle tissue of any animal–beef, lamb, veal, mutton, pork or poultry. 'Organ meats' of 'ofal' is the term used for non-muscle tissue such as liver, kidneys, etc.

Most muscle meat is about 20% protein, 10–30% fat, and the remainder water.

Meat Bar. Dehydrated cooked meat and fat; a modern form of pemmican.

Meat Conditioning. After an animal has been slaughtered, muscle glycogen breaks down to lactice acid, which tends to improve the texture and keeping qualities of the meat. Meat that has been left until these changes have taken place is 'conditioned'.

Meat, Curing. Pickling with the aid of sodium chloride, sodium nitrate and some sodium nitrite, which permits the growth of only salt-tolerant bacteria and inhibits the growth of Clostridium botulinum. The nitrite is the effective preserving agent and the nitrate. Its converted into nitrite during the process. The red colour occur due to the formation of nitrosomyoglobin from the myoglobin and nitric oxyde.

Meat Extract. Refers to the water-soluble part of meat that is mainly responsible for flavour. Commercially is made during the manufacture of corned beaf; minced meat is immersed in boiling water, when the water-soluble extractives are partially leached out. This 'soup' is concentrated and produced the meat extract (so-called No. 1 extract) of commerce. (Exhaustive extraction of the meat produces 'Direct Extract', containing more gelatin).

It is rich in the B vitamins (particularly B_2, nicotinic acid and B_{12}), meat bases and potasiu. Shown by Pavlov that meat extract is the most powerful oral stimulant of gastic acid secretion.

Medicinal Paraffin. A mineral oil having no nutritive value as it is not affective by digestive enzymes and passes through the intestine unchanged. It finds use as a mind laxative because of its lubricant properties if taken at the same time as the fat-soluble vitamins, these go into solution in the oil and pass through the digestive tract unabsorbed.

Melampyrin. Dulcitol.

Melangeur. Mixing vessel having rollers riding on a rotating horizontal bed. Used to mix substances of pasty consistency (hence meltangeuring).

Melezitose. Trisaccharide which is composed of two glucose and one fructose; hydrolysed to glucose puls the disaccharide turanose (3-α-D-glucoside-D-fructose).

Melibiose. Disaccharide, 6(α–D galactoside)-D-glucose.

Mellorine. US term for ice-cream made from non-butter fat.

Membrane, Semi-permeable. One that allows the passage of small but not large molecules: *e.g.* pig's bladder is permeable to water but not salt; collodion is permeable to salt but not protein molecules. The exchange of water and salts between tissue of the body and red blood cells is possible because of the semi-permeable nature of the walls.

Menadione. Obsolete term for vitamin K_3, 2-methyl-1, 4-naphthoquinone.

Menaquino. 2-methyl-1, 4-naphthoquinone, genric descriptor of substances with vitamin K activity, formerly called menadione.

Mercapturic Acid. Complex of cysteine with naphthalene or various halogenated aromatic hydrocarbons (such as bromobenzene) whereby the latter compounds get detoxiated and excreted in the urine.

Meringues. Confections made by beating together a mixture of sugar and white of eggs.

Mesomorph. Description given to a well-covered individual with well- developed muscles.

Mesophiles. Micro-organisms that grow best at temperatures between 25 and 40C, usually with not grow at temperature below 5C.

Metabolic Rate. Rate of utilisation of energy.

Metabolism. Refers to the process of chemical change that goes on in living cells: growth of new tissues, breakdown of old tissue, production of energy. Anabolism is building up and catabolism is breaking down. Intermediary metabolism describes the biochemical stages in the changes of, for example, glucose to carbon dioxide and water.

Metalloproteins. Proteins linked to a metal, like hemoglobin, cytochrome, peroxidase, ferritin, siderophilin, all of which contain iron, and chlorocruorin, which contain copper.

Metaproteins. Refers to the products of the action on proteins of dilute acids or alkalies, they are no longer soluble at their isoelectric points but are soluble in weak acid or alkali.

Methaemoglobin. Oxidised form of hemoglobin (unlike oxyhemoglobin, which is a loose and reversible combination with oxygen) which cannot transport oxygen to the tissues. Present in small quantities in normal blood, increased after certain drugs and after smoking, found rarely as congenital abnormality.

Can be formed in blood of babies after consumption of small amounts of nitrate found naturally in vegetables grown in certain areas and in some drinking water, because the lace of acidity in the stomach permits reduction of nitrate to nitrite.

Methionine. An essential amino acid; one of the three containing sulphur–cystine, cysteine and methionine.

Methionine is available on the commercial scale and is added to animal feeds, where it is often, but not always, the limiting amino acid.

Chemically, aminomethylthiol butyric acid.

Methionine Sulphoximine. Substance which is formed by reaction between nitrogen trichloride ('agene') and the amino acid methionine when flour is treated with a gene as a bleaching agent. Causes running fits in dogs, toxic to man.

Methylated Spirits. Ethyl alcohol having methyl alcohol, coloured with a dye and given a repulsive small by the addition of pyridine. It toxicity occurs due to the presence of the methyl alcohol.

Methylene Blue. Blue dye that becomes colourless when reduced, the so-called leuco-form. It finds use in cell respiration experiments to indicate when oxygen is being consumed.

Methylene Blus Dye-reduction Test. When methylene blue or resazurin is added to milk, the bacteria present take up oxygen and change the colour of the dye.

Methylene blue become colourless; resazurin changes blue-purple-pink-while.

The speed of the change indicates the bacterial content. Pasteurised milk must not reduce dye in half an hour.

Methyl-histidine. (3-methylhistidine). Found in animal muscle; suggested as analytical method of measuring meat content of products.

Meulengracht Diet. For peptic ulcer patients; sieved foods like meat, chicken vegetables, at 2-hourly intervals. Differs from Sippy and Lenhartz diets in being much richer in protein. The intention has been to neutralise the acid in the stomach by the buffering effect of the protein.

Micro-aerophiles. Micro-organism that can grow in low concentrations of oxygen and so lead to spoilage of foodstuffs unless all oxygen is excluded.

Microbiological Assay. Biological assay which is using micro-organisms; used fat vitamins and amino acids in particular. The principal is that the organism gets inoculated into a medium containing all the needed growth factors except the one under examination; the rate of growth is then proportional to the amount of this particular factor added in the test substance. Rate of growth is then proportional to the amount of this particular factor added in the test substance. Rate of growth determined by turbidity or by titrating the acid produced after 2–3 days incubation.

Microencapsulation. Preparation of small particles of solids or droplets of liquids inside thin polymeric coatings (ranging from beeswax and starch to gelatin and polyacrylic acid). The microcapsules range from tenths to thousandth of microns is size and find use to prepare liquid as free-flowing powers or compressed solids, to separate reactive materials, reduce toxicity, protect against oxidation and control rate of release; used for enzymes, flavours nutrients, etc.

Microgram. One-thousandth part of a milligram; symbol μg.

Micron. One-thousandth of a millimetre; unit of measurement of bacterial size.

Micronisation. Extremely rapid heating with infrared radition produced by heating propane on a ceramic tile or with nichrome wire elements.

Microoganisms. Generally this term refers to bacteria, moulds and yeasts, of interest in food spoilage, as causes of disease, of value in food preservation and processing and as foodstuffs themselves (termed single cell protein).

Microwave Heating. Irradiation.

Milk. Refers to the secretion of the mammary gland of animals including cow, buffalo, goat, ass, mare, ewe and camel.

Cow's milk is especially rich in calcium (1.2g per litre), and riboflavin (2mg per litre) and contains per litre 47g lactose, 33g protein, 38g fat, 500μg vitamin A (as both retinol and carotene), 0.4 mg thiamin, 0.8mg niacin, 50μg folate, 0.3μg vitamin D, about 15mg vitamin C, and small amounts of other B vitamins and minerals. Jersey, Guernsay, South Devon and Channel Islands milk contain about 48g fat.

Buffalo Milk–75g fat, 43g protein and 45g carbohydrate per litre.

Milk, Accredited. Referred to milk untreated by heat, from cows examined at specific intervals for freedom from disease.

Milk Acidophilus. A preparation which is similar to cultured butter-milk but soured by Lactobacillus instead of acid-producing streptococci.

Milk-alkali Syndrome. Weakness and lethargy caused by prolonged adherence to a diet rich in milk (more than 2 pints) per day and alkalies.

Milk, Buddeised. Milk which is preserved by the addition of hydrogen peroxide.

Milk, Citrated. Milk to which sodium citrate has been added to combine with the calcium and inhibit the curdling of caseinogen which would normally occur in the stomach.

Milk, Designated. Legally milk is designated pasteurised or sterilised and also tuberculin tested.

The special designation 'accredited' has been abolished.

Milk, Dried. Milk that is evaporated to dryness, usually by spray or roller-drying. May be whole or full-cream milk (26% fat), three quarter cream (not less than 20% fat), half-cream (not less than 14% fat), quarter-cream (not less than 8% fat) or skim milk (1% fat).

Milk, Dye-reduction Test. Methylene blue dye-reduction test.

Milk, Evaporated. Concentrated to about 45% of its original volume by evaporation. Also termed as unsweetened, condensed milk.

Milk Fat Test. Gerber test.

Milk, Filled. Milk from which the natural fat has been removed and replaced with fat from another source.

Milk, Freezing-point Test. The sample of milk is cooled below its freezing point and seeded with a crystal of ice. The temperature rises to the freezing point (FP) of milk as the whole freezes–normally–0.530 to–0.560C.

When milk has been adulterated, the FP rises nearer to that of water. FPs above–0.530C are indicative of adulteration.

Milk, Frozen or Fresh Frozen. Milk gets pasteurised, treated with an ultrasonic vibrator at 5 million cycles per second for 5 minutes and frozen to 10F. It will keep for a year, and when thawed gets indistinguishable from the original milk.

Milk, Half-cream. Refers to dried milk power in which the fat content gets reduced to half for infant feeding, particularly for premature infants.

Milk, Homogenised. Mechanical treatment breaks up and redistributes the fat globules throughout the milk to prevent the cream rising to the surface.

Milk, Humanised. Cow'milk that has had its composition modified to resemble human milk. The main change is a reduction in protein content often achieved by dilution with carbohydrate and restoration of the fat content.

Milk, Irradiated. Milk that is subjected to ultraviolet light, when the 7-dehydrocholesterol present naturally is partly converted into vitamin D.

Milk, Lactose-hydrolysed. Milk, in which the lactose is hydrolysed go glucose and galactose by treatment with the enzymen lactase, intended for infants who are lactase-deficient.

Milks, Fermented. In various countries milk, from the ass, mare, cow, goat and buffalo, is fermented with a mixture of bacteria and yeasts, when the lactose gets converted to lactic acid and, in some drinks, to alcohol. These fermented milks include busa (Turkestan), cieddu (Italy), Dadh (India), kefir (Balkans), Kumiss (Steppes), laban Zabadi (Egypt), mazun (Armenia), taette (N. Europe), skyr (Iceland), mast (Iran), crowdies (Scotland), kuban and yoghurt.

Milk-stone. Deposit of calcium and magnesium phosphates, protein, etc. which are produced when milk is heated to temperatures above 60C.

Milk, Sweetened, Condensed. Evaporated to less than one third volume and sugar added as preservative; may be full cream or skimmed.

Milk, Toned. Dried, skim milk added to a high-fat milk such as buffalo milk, to reduce the fat content but maintain the total solids. If the fat were diluted simply by adding water, the milk would not be 'toned up'.

Milk, TT. Tuberculin tested. Applied to milk from herd that has been attested free from tubercle by a veterinary inspector.

Milk, Turbidity Test. In order to distinguish sterilised milk from pasteurised. During sterilisation, the milk is held at 104–116C from 20–40 minutes, when all the albumin gets precipitated. In the test the filtrate from an ammonium sulphate precipitation should remain clear on heating, indicating that no albumin was present in solution and the milk had therefore been strilised.

Millerator. Wheat-cleaning machine which is consisting of two sieves, the upper one retaining particles larger than wheat, the lower one rejecting particles smaller that wheat.

Millet. Cereal of a number of species of Graminease smaller that wheat and rice and high in fibre content.

Common millet (Panicum and Setaria species) also known as China, Italian, Indian, French hog, proso, panicled and broom corn millet; grow very raiply, 2–21/2 months from sowing to harvest.

Milling. Refers to the conversion of cereal grain into its derivative–*e.g.* wheat into flour, brown rice to white rice.

Million's Test. For proteins; actually a test for the hydroxyphyenyl group and therefore for tyrosine, but sine every protein contains some tyrosine, it is used as a general protein test.

The reagent consists of mercury in nitric acid and gives a white precipitate with proteins which turns red on heating.

Milt. Refers to the soft roe of the male fish. Also the name given to the spleen of animals.

Miltone. A toned milk developed in India in which peanut protein is added to buffalo or cow's milk to extend supplies.

Mincemenut. 30% dried fruit and peel 30% sugar, 2.5% fat, 0.5 acertic acid, not less than 65% soluble solids.

In America a heavily spiced mixture of chopped meat, apples and raisins.

Mineralocorticoids. Obsolescent term for the steriod hormones of the adrenal cortex which control the excretion of salt and water by the kidney.

Mineral Salts. Refers to the inorganic salts, including sodium, potassium, calcium, chloride, phosphate, sulphate, etc.

Mineral Waters. The term used for the natural, untread, spring water, some of which are naturally carbonated, may be slightly alkaline or salty.

The term is also applied to artificially carbonated water, 'soda water' or club soda.

Miners'Cramp. Cramp which occur due to loss of salt from the body caused by excessive seating, occurs in tropical climates and with severe exercise–mining often combines the two. Prevented by consuming salt, *e.g.,* salt tablets in the tropics and for athlete.

Minifoods. Name assigned to single cell proteins.

Minisata Disease. Poisoning due to an organic form of mercury (methyl mercury) named after Minimata Bay in Japan, where fish containing mercury from contamination caused such poisoning.

Mint. Many varieties of the species Mentha–spearmint, M. spicata, peppermint, M. piperita. It is used to flavour meat, fish, tobacco, etc.

Oil of peppermint is distilled from stem and leaves of M. piprita, and used both pharmaceutically and as a flavour.

Miotin. Unidentified urinary excretion product of biotin, together with triotin and rhiotin.

Mirepoix. Bed of vegetables which are used to give flavour to braised meats and also soups and sauces.

Miso. Old Japanese food which is prepared by fermentation of mouldy rice of koji (Aspergillus) with soya bean and salt.

Mixograph. An American instrument which is used for measuring the physical properties of a dough, similar in principle to the farmograph, which see.

Molasses. Residue which is left after repeated crystallisation of sugar, contains sucrose, glucose and fructose and (if from beet) raffinose and small quantities of dextrans, will crystallise, 67% sucrose, 260 kcal (1.1MJ) per 100g: contains more than 500mg iron per 100g with traces of other minerals.

Molisch Reaction. A test for carbohydrates. The reagent is a 5% solution of alpha-naphthol in alcohol; two drops added to the test solution and concentrated sulphuric acid poured down the side of the tube to form a lower layer. Violet zone is formed at the junction.

Molybdenum. A constituent of at least two mammalian enzymes–namely xanthine oxidase and aldehyde dehydrogenase–and therefore it is a dietary essential for man, although dietary deficiencies are never encountered. Excess is toxic.

Monellin. Refers to the active sweet principle, a protein, from the serendipity berry, Dioscoreophyllum cumminsii, 1500-3000 times as sweet as sucrose.

Monophaiga. Desire for one type of food.

Monosaccharides. Group name of the simplest sugars, including those composed of 3 carbon atoms (trioses), 4 (tetroses), 5 (pentoses), 6 (hexoses) and 7 (heptoses). Also known as monoses or monosaccharoses.

Moreton Bay Bug. Or Bay lobster, a variety of sand lobster found in Australia.

Mother of Vinegar. Vinegar.

Mottled Teeth. In areas where the drinking water is having fluoride at a level of several parts per million, dull, chalky patches occur one the teeth known as motling. These teeth are relatively free decay, and lower levels of fluoride, about 1ppm, reduce decay without causing molting.

Mould Bran. A fungal amylase preparation which is produce by growing mould on moist wheat bran, used as source of starch-splitting enzymes.

Moulds. Fungi which are characterised by their branched filamentous structure of mycelium:

1. They can being about food spoilage very rapidly–white Mucor, grey-green Penicillium black Aspergillus–and produce mycotoxins.
2. Used for large-scale production of citric acid (Aspergillusniger), ripening of cheese (species of Penicillium) and as source of enzymes for used in the food industry.
3. Mushrooms belong to this family of fungi.
4. A number of foods are fermented with moulds, *e.g.*, idli, miso and tempeh.
5. The mycelium of Fusarium species is used as a manufactured food tempeh.
6. Most of the antibiotics have been mould products.

Mucin. Naturally occurring complex of protein and

carbohydrates, highly viscous.

Mucopolysaccharides. Group of polysaccharides which are containing as amino sugar and uronic acid, constitute of mucoproteins of cartilage tendons, connective tissue, cornea, heparin and blood group substances.

Mucoproteins. Refers to the members of the group of glycoproteins containing a sugar, usually chondroitin sulphate, combined with amino acids or peptides; occur in mucin secreted in the stomach, saliva and various glands.

Mucosa. Name given to the moist tissue lining, for example, the mouth (buccal mucosa), intestines and respiratory tract.

The intestinal wall in having two sides, the inner, or mucosal, side, and the outer, or serosal, side.

Mulberry. Morus nigra (also white mulberry, M. alba). Of little commercial importance.

Multipurpose Food. Indian multipurpose food is made from peanut flour and chickpea flour with calcium carbonate, and vitamins A, B_1 and B_2 and is having 40% protein.American multipurpose food is based on soya.

Muscarine. Refers to quaternary trimethylammonium salt of 2-methyl-3hydroxy-5-(aminomethyl)-tetrahydrofuran. It is the toxic material is red variety of the mushroom Amanita muscaria, the fly fungus and other fungi.

Muscle. The contractile cellular unit of skeletal muscle is the fibre. This is a long cylinder in shape and composed of many myofibrils. Chemically, the muscle fibre is composed of three proteins myosin, action and tropomyosin.

Muscle Adenylic Acid. Adenosine-5-phosphoric acid, yeast adenylic acid is adenosine-3-phosphoric acid.

Mushroom. Agaricus campestris.

Mashroom Sugar. Trehalose.

Mussel. Mytilus edulis. Bivalave, cultivated at 25-50 tons per acre, yield 6-10 tons wet weight of mean per acre, take 4 years to reach marketable size–5cm, 20% of weight is meat.

Mustard. Powdered seed of black or brown mustard (Brassica nigra or B. Juncea) mixed with yellow or white (Sinapisi alba). Active principles are glycosides–singigrin to black, sinalbin in white. When moistened, the enzyme myrosinase liberated the characteristically flavoured oil.

English mustard : having not more than 10% wheat flour and water.

Dijon mustard : made exclusively from B. nigra or B. juncea with vinegar, grapel juice or wine, and not coloured.

Violet mustard : coloured with grape juice.

French mustard : coloured mustard, vinegar, salt, turmeric, cayenne pepper, cloves, pimento.

Mustard leaves eaten raw in salads (mustard and cress are seed leaves of S. alba); much of the commercial product is a strain of rape (Brassica napus), a different strain from that used for edible oil.

Mustard Oil. Used as cooking at in Bengal and Bigar. The seeds are often contaminated with seeds of Argemone mexicana, which is having an alkaloid, argemone oil. The contaminated mustard oil has been the cause of epidemic dropsy, as the sanguinarine inhibits the oxidation of pyruvic acid which gets accumulated in the blood.

Mutagen. A substance that is able to produce genetic damage by affecting spermatozoa or ova.

Mutton. Meat of sheep older than 1 year.

Mycelial Protein. Name given to mould mycelium prepared as foodstuff. Fusarium species and Neuraspora species grown on carbohydrate have been used.

Mycotoxins. Refers to toxins which are formed by fungi (moulds) especially Aspergillus flavours under tropical conditions and Pencillum and Fusarium species under tropical conditions and Pencillum and Fusarium species under temperate conditions. The problem is created by the storage of food under damp conditions which favour the growth of the moulds.

Myocardial Infraction. Refers to the damage to heart

muscle due to failure of the blood supply to the muscle (ischaremia).

Myogen. Refers to the protein of muscle. It is about 20% of the total; and albumin, not present in the muscle fibrils but oly in the sarcoplasm in which the fibrils are embedded.

Myoglobin. Refers to a complex protein in muscle which is similar to the hemoglobin of the blood (but one-fourth of its molecular weight). It is composed of the iron-containing pigment haem and the protein globin. It serves as a storage mechanism for oxygen for the cells, as it can reversily add oxygen to from oxymyglobin. The globin is denatured by heat to a brown pigment; hence the change from the red colour of raw meat to brown on cooking. When meat is cured with nitrite, the myoglobin or nitrosomyoglobin.

Myosin. Major fraction which is about two-fifths, of muscle protein. A globulin which is insoluble in water but soluble in salt solution. Combines with the protein actin to form actomyosin; the complex dissociates in the presence of ATP.

Myristic Acid. A long-chain saturated fatty acid, $CH_3(CH_2)_{12}COOH$. Occurs as triglyceride in nutmeg, coconut butter, lard, spermaceti and wool wax.

Myrosinase. Glysidase enzyme in mustard seed that hydrolyses myrosin or sinigrin to glucose and ally; isothiocyanate (mustard oil).

N

Natto. Fermented soya bean (Japan).

Neats Food. Ox or calf's foot which is used for making soups and jellies. Now called cow's heels.

Neat's-foot Oil. Oil obtained from the knuckle bones of cattle. It is used in lather working and for canning sardines.

NEO-DHC. Neohesperidin dihydrochalcone; non nutritive sweetener.

Neohesperidin dihydrochalcone. 1000 times as sweet as sucrose. It is formed by hydrogenation of naturally occurring flavonoid neohesperidin.

Neomycin. Refers to antibiotic isolated 1049 from Streptomyces fradii. It is used to some extent in controlling infections in food processing.

Neroli Oil. Prepared from blossoms of the bitter orange by steam distillation. Yellowish oil with intense odour of orange blossom.

Nescafe. Trade name (Nestles Ltd) for a dried instant coffee. Contains more potassium than any other food–5.5%.

Nessler Reagent. Refers to an alkaline solution of the double iodide of mercury and potassium. Gives an orange-brown with ammonia and used for quantitative estimation.

Net Dietary Protein Calories. Net dietary protein energy ratio.

Net dietary protein Energy Ratio. Refers to the protein

content of diet or food expressed as protein energy multiplied by net protein utilisation (which) divided by total energy.

Before the change from calories to joules this was called dietary protein calories per cent, NDpcal%.

Net protein Utilisation. Refers to the measure of quality of protein in terms of amount of dietary protein retained in the body under specified experimental conditions. Previously expressed as percentage, i.g. egg protein and human milk had NPU 100; wheat protein 50. Now expressed as ratio 1.0 and 0.5, respectively.

By convention measured at 10% dietary protein level, NPU [illegible] t which level the protein synthetic mechanism in the growing animal can use all the protein so long as the balance of amino acids is correct. When fed at 4% dietary protein level, said to be that level which the NPU is maximum, the value is termed NPU standardised. If the food or diet get fed as it is, i.e., not incorporated into a diet with other ingredients, the value is NPU operative (NPUop).

Net Protein Value. Produce of net protein utilisation and protein content per cent.

Neuberg Ester. Name assigned to fructose-6 phosphate, one of the intermediates in glucose metabolism.

Neuraminic Acid. Sialic acid.

Neurine. Trimethylvinylammonium hydroxide which is formed during putrefaction by dehydration of choline and also occurred in egg yolk, brain and bile; toxic.

New Zealand process. A drying process which is applied to meat. It is immersed in hot oil under vacuum, when it dries to 3% moisture in about 4 hours. The fat is removed from the dry meat in a hydroextractor.

NFE. Nitrogen-free. extract. In the analysis of foods and animal feeding stuffs this fraction is having the sugars and starches plus small amount of other materials.

Niaein. Generic descriptor for pyridine-3 carboxylic acid and derivatives exhibiting qualitatively the biological activity of nicotinamide. The term nicotinic acid refers specifically to pyridine-3 carboxylic acid; its amide is nicotinamide.

Niacinogens. Name assigned to protein-niacin complexes found in cereals.

Niactyin. Refers to the bound forms of the vitamin niacin which are found in some foods, particularly cereals. Complexes of niacin with polysaccharides of cellulose type and peptide or glycopeptide; not hydrolysed by intestinal enzymes, so biologically unavailable, but can be liberated by acid or alkaline hydrolysis or by baking the cereal, especially with an alkaline baking powder.

Nickel. Present in foods and in animal and human tissues. It is not essential for plants or animals but improves growth of many plants. Metallic nickel finds use as catalyst in hydrogenation of fast.

Nicotinamide. Nicotinic acid.

Nicotinamide Adenine Dinucleotide (NAD). Refers to the complex of nicotinamide with adenine, two molecules of ribose and two molecules of phosphate. Also known as Coenzyme I, diphosphopyridine nucleotide (DPN) cozymase and as Euler's yeast coenzyme. It is essential part of the mechanism of oxidation in the tissues.

Nicotinamide Adenine Dinucleotide Phosphate (NADP). Complex of nicotinamide with two molecules of ribose, adenine and three molecules of phosphate. Also called triphosphopyridine nucleotide (TPN), coenzyme II and Warburg and Christian's coenzyme. Essential part, along with NAD, of the mechanism of oxidation in the tissues.

Nicotinamide Nucleotides. Nicotinamide adenine dinucleotide (NAD) and nicotinamide adenine dinucleotide phosphate (NADP) has been common carriers of hydrogen and electrons in oxidation and reduction reactions.

Nicotinate, Sodium. Sodium salt of nicotinic acid. It is used, among other purposes, to preserve the red colour in fresh and processed meats.

Night Blindness. Nyctalopia. Inability to see in dim light through deficiency of vitamin A. Dark-adaptation test find use as an index of vitamin A deficiency, as night blindness is the first symptom.

Ninhydrin Test. From proteins and amino acids (actually for the amino group). Pink, purple or blue colour gets developed on reacting the amino acid or peptide with ninhydrin (triketohydrindene hydrate).

Nioigome. Perfumed rice.

Nisin. Antibiotic which was isolated 1944 from lactice streptococci group N. Non-toxic, polypeptide, inhibits some but not all clostridia, not used medically. The only antibiotic permitted in many countries in food preservation (in certain foods). It is naturally present in cheese, being produces by a number of strains of cheese starter organisms. It is used to prolong storage life of cheese, milk, cream, soups, canned frits and vegetables, canned fish and milk pudding. Used at 2–4μg per g of processed cheese and 1–5μg per g of canned peas. It also lowers the resistance of many thermophilic bacteria to heat and so permits a reduction in the time and/or temperature of heating in the processing of canned vegetables.

Nitrate. Natural constituent of plants, beets, rhubarb, cabbage, broccoli, cauliflower can contain up to 1 mg/kg. Within one or two days after harvesting, some of the nitrate is converted into nitrite. It finds use together with nitrite in pickling of meats and is converted into nitrite in the process. Nitrites can react with hemoglobin to form methaemoglobin (which see), especially in young infants, and an upper limit of 45–50 mg nitrate per litre drinking water has been recommended for infants.

Nitrites. Found in many plant foods, since they are rapidly formed by the reduction of naturally occurring nitrate. Nitrite has been the essential agent in preserving meat by pickling, since it inhibits the growth of clostridia, it also combines with the myoglobin of meat of form the characteristic red nitrosomyoglobin.

Nitrogen. In nutrition the term 'nitrogen' is used to refer to ammonium salts and nitrates as plant fertilisers, to proteins and amino acids as animal nutrients, and to urea and ammonium salts as excretory products. In other words, all nitrogen- containing substances are loosely referred to as 'nitrogen'.

Nitrogen Balance. Refers to the difference between the dietary intake of nitrogen (as protein) and its excretion (as urea and other waste products).

During growth and tissue repair (convalescence) the body has been in positive N balance, i.e. ingestion is greater than loss. In fevers, fasting and wasting diseases the loss is greater than the intake, and the individual is in negative balance.

Healthy adults are excreting the same amount as is being ingested and so are N equilibrium.

Nitrogen Trichloride. As bread 'improver'.

Nitrosamines. Refers to the group of compounds bearing the nitroso group on the N of the corresponding amimes– N- nitrosodimethylamine, N- nitrosodiethylamine, occur in amounts of a few micrograms per kg in mushrooms, fermented fish meal and smoked fish, and in pickled food by reaction between nitrite and secondary amines. Causes cancer in all species of animals examined.

Nitrosomyoglobin. Refers to the red colour of cured meat. It gets formed by the reaction of nitric oxide from the pickling salts (saltpetre) with the muscle pigment, myoglobin. Fades in light to yellow-brown metmyoglobin.

Nitrous Oxide. A gas which is used as a propellant in pressurised containers, e.g. to eject cream or salad dressing from containers.

Noggin. Used as a measure of liquor + ¼ pint, also known as a quartern.

Non-esterified Fatty Acids. Refer to free fatty acids in the blood, about 10% of the total blood fatty acids, usually 0.5 – 1.0 micromole per litre.

Non-pareils. The silver beads used to decorate confectioner, made from sugar coated with silver foil or aluminium–copper alloy.

Noradrenaline. Hormone which is secreted by the adrenal medulla together with adrenaline (which see), also known as norepinephrine. Physiological effects similar to those of adrenaline, chemically differs only by the loss of amethyl group.

Nordihydroguaiaretic Acid (NDGA). Refers to the substance of plant origin (the creosote bush) used as an antioxidant for fats.

Norite. Refers to the activated carbon used to decolorise solutions.

Nougat. Sweetmeat made from a mixture of gelatin or egg albumin with sugar and starch syrup, and the whole thoroughly aerated.

Nubbing. Term used in the canning industry for 'toping and tailing' of gooseberries.

Nucellar Layer. Of wheat, the layer cells that surrounds the endosperm and protects it from the entry of moisture.

Nucieic Acids. Combined with proteins they form the nucleoproteins of cell nuclei. There are two main types of nucleic acid : ribonucleic acid (RNA), consisting of phosphoric acid, two purines (adenine and guanine), two pyrimidines (cytosine and uracil) and the sugar ribose; and desoxyribonucleic acid (DNA), which differs in containing desoxyribose as the sugar, and thymine in place of uracil.

RNA and DNA play a key role in the synthesis of proteins in the body and in the transmission of hereditary characteristics.

Nucleoproteins occur in some foods such as fish roe, and are useful as a source of protein, but they are not essential to the diet and the nucleic acids are readily synthesised in the body.

Nucleo-albuminate, Iron. A preparation of iron and casein. It also called of both plants and animals.

Nucleosides. Compound of purine or pyrimidine base with sugar. For example, adenine plus ribose forms adenosine–the nucleoside. With the addition of phosphoric acid a nucleotide is formed.

Necleotides. Compound of purine or pyrimidine base with sugar and phosphoric acid.

Nuoc Mam. Refers to the permented fish sauce from Vietnam and Cambodia. The fish is digested by autolytic enzymes in the presence of added salt to inhibit bacteria.

Nutrients. Essential dietary factors like vitamins, minerals, amino acids and facts. Sources of energy are not termed nutrients so that a commonly used phase is 'energy and nutrients' (calories and nutrients).

Nutrification. A term which is used of the addition of nutrients to foods at such a level as to make a major contribution to the diet.

Nutrition. Refers to the study of foods in relation to the needs of living organisms.

Nutritive Ratio. Refers to the measure of the value of a feeding ration for growth (or milk production) compared with its fattening value. It is the sum of the digestible carbohydrate, protein and 2.3 × fat, divided by digestible protein. (Calorie value of fat is 2.3 times carbohydrate and protein.) Ratio 4–5 for growth, 7–8 for fattening.

Nutritive Value Index. Term used in animal feeding; intake of digestible energy expressed as energy digestibility multiplied by voluntary intake of dry matter of a particular feed divided by metabolic weight (weight to the power of 0.75), compared with standard feed.

Nutro-Biscuit. Biscuit which is baked from a mixture of 60% wheat flour and 40% peanut flour–contains 16–17% protein; developed in India.

Nutro-Macaroni. Refers to the mixture of 80 parts wheat flour, 20 parts defeated peanut meal (total 19% protein); developed in India.

Nyctalopia. Night blindness.

O

Oestrogens. Female sex hormones. There are two groups, oestrone and oestradiol, which stimulate the ovaries, and progesterone, produced by the corpus luteum, which stimulates the uterus.

Synthetic hormones include ethinyl oestradiol, stilboestrol and hexoestrol. The latter two find use in chemical caponisation of cockerels, by implantation under the skin, and to increase the growth rate of cattle, by implantation during the last 3 months before slaughter.

Oestrone. Refers to one of the female sex hormones.

Offal. Corruption of 'off-fall'. With reference to meat, the term includes all parts that are cut away when the carcass gets dressed, including liver, kidneys, brain spleen, pancreas, thymus, tripe and tongue. In the USA the term used is 'organ meats'.

With reference to cereals, offals have been the bran and germ discarded when milling to a white flour.

Oilseed. A wide variety of seeds are grown as a source of oils, e.g., cottonseed, sesame, groundnut, sunflower, soya, palm, etc. After extraction of the oil the residue is a valuable source of protein, the so-called seed cake.

Oils, Essential. Essential Oils.

Oils, Fixed. Refers to the triglycerides, the edible oils, as distinct from the volatile or essential oils.

Okra. Also known as gumbo, bamya, bamies and ladies'

fingers (Hibiscus esculentus). Small ridged mucilaginous pods resembling a small cucumber. It is used in soups and stews.

Oleandomycin. Antibiotic is sometimes used as additive to chicken feed.

Oleic Acid. Refers to the long-chain fatty acid with total of 18 carbon atoms; unsaturated with one double bond, 2–octadecenoic acid; found in most fats; high percentage in human fat, and butter. By far the most abundant of the unsaturated acids.

Oleoresins. In the preparation of some spices like pepper, ginger and capsicum, the aromatic material is extracted with solvents which are evaporated off, leaving behind thick oily products called oleoresins.

Oilgodynamic. Sterilising effect of traces of certain metals. For example, silver in concentration of 1 in 5 million will kill Escherichia coli and staphylococci in 3 hours.

Oligosaccharides. Carbohydrates which are composed of 3–10 monosaccharide units (with more than 10 units they are termed polysaccharides).

Olive. Fruit of evergreen tree, Oleo europea, picked unripe when green or ripe when they have turned dark blue or purplish, and usually pickled in brine.

Olive oil, obtained by pressing the ripe fruits, find use in cooking, as salad oil and for canning sardines. It is one of the few vegetable oils to have only small amounts of polyunsaturated fatty acids.

Omophagia. Eating of raw or uncooked food.

Oncotic Pressure. The osmotic pressure of colloids. Blood plasma has an oncotic pressure of 28mm of mercury.

Onion. Bulb of allium cepa. Analysis of mature bulb per g : 93g water, 5g sugars, 1g protein, 23 kcal (100kJ), 3-15mg vitamin C.

Opsomania. Craving for special food.

Optical Activity. Refers to the ability of certain substances like sugars and acids to rotate the plane of polarised light. If the plane of light is rotated to the right, the substance is dextrorotatory and is designeated by the prefix (+), if laevorotatory, the prefix is (–). A mixture of the two forms is optically inactive and is termed racemic.

Optical Rotation. Optical activity.

Orange. Fruit of citrus sinensis. Of nutritive value mainly due to its vitamin C content. The juice has the same composition.

Analysis per 100g : carbohydrate 8.5g, protein 0.6g, kcal 32 (150kj), Ca 40mg, Fe 0.3mg, carotene 50ug, vitamin C 40-60mg.

Blood oranges are coloured by the presence of anthocyanins (cyanidin-3-glucoside and delphinidin-3-glucoside) in the juice vesicles.

Orange Butter. Chopped whole orange cooked, sweetened and homogenised.

Orange Colours. Orange G-disodium salt of 1-pthenylazo-2-naphthol-6,8-disulphonic acid. Stable to reducing agents.

Orange RN-sodium salt of 1-sulphylazo-2naphthol-6-phenolic acid.

Orange-flower Water. Neroli oil is prepared from the flowers of the bitter orange by steam distillation. The condensed water layer from the distillation is orange-flower water.

Orange Oil. The peel oil, 90% limonene, main odoriferous constituent n-decylic aldehyde (decanal), also linalool and nonylic alcohol. Oil of bitter orange is similar but is having a glucoside that confers that bitterness.

Orchil. Red colour which is obtained from lichens of the Roccella species; legally permitted in food in most countries. Colouring principle is orcin (dihydroxy toluene) and orcein, slightly soluble in water to give wine-red solution, yellower with acid, blue with alkalies.

Organoleptic. Affecting a bodily organ or sense, used particularly of the combination of taste (perceived in the mouth) and aroma (perceived in the nose). There are four tastes—acid, bitter, salt and sweet, with the additional aspect of astrigency.

Ornithine. An amino acid that is part of the urea cycle, not of nutritional importance, because it is not found in protein food-stuffs.

Ornithine-arginine Cycle. Urea cycle.

Orotic Acid. Uracil-4-carboxylic acid, and intermediate in the biosynthesis of pyrimidines; a growth factor for certain microorganisms and called vitamin B_{13}.

Ortanique. Citrus fruit, cross between orange and tangerine.

Oryzenin. The major protein of rice. It is classed as one of the glutelins.

Osmosis. Passages through a semi-permeable membrane.

Osmosis, Reverse. Refers to the passage of water from a more concentrated to a less concentrated solution through a semipermeable memberane by the application of pressure. Used for desalination of sea-water, concentration of fruit juices and processing of cheese whey. Membranes commonly cellulose acetate or polyamide.

Osmotic pressure. The attractive power exerted by a solution for water molecules. Usually demonstrated by placing a solution of a salt in a vessel separated by a semi-permeable membrane (e.g., pig's bladder) from pure water. Water passes across the membrane to dilute the salt solution until the hydrostatic pressure of the solution counterbalances the attractive power of the solution for the water, i.e., its osmotic pressure.

Ossein. Organic structure of the bone which is left behind when the mineral salts are removed by solution in dilute acid. Chemically it is similar to collagen and hydrolysed by boiling water to gelatin, hence the manufacture of glue from bones-know as ossein gelatin.

Osseomucoid. Muccid substance which is forming part of the structure of bone.

Osteomalacia. Bone disorder in adults equivalent to rickets in children; due to shortage of vitamin D giving rise to inadequate absorption of calcium and loss of calcium from the bones.

Ovaltine. The albumin of egg-white; comprises 55% of the total solids.

Ovaltine. Trade name (A. Wander Ltd.) for a preparation of malt extract, milk, eggs, cocoa and soya, for consumption as a beverage when added to milk. Fortified with vitamin B, vitamin D and nicotinic acid.

Oven Spring. Refers to the sudden increases in the volume of dough during the first 10-12 minutes of baking-due to increased rate of fermentation and to expansion of gases.

Overrun. Term used in ice-cream manufacture-the percentage increase in the volume of the mi: caused by the beating-in or air. Optimum overrun, 70-100%. To prevent excessive aeration United States regulations state that ice cream must weigh 405lb per gallon.

Ovoflavin. Name given to substance which is isolated from eggs, shown to be identical with riboflavin.

Ovomucin. A carbohydrate-protein complex in egg-white, 1-3% of the total solids. Responsible for the firmness of egg-white.

Ovomucoid. Refers to a protein of egg-white, 12% of the total solids. Acts as a specific inhibitor of the digestive enzyme trypsin, but gets destroyed by the stomach enzyme pepsin.

Oxalic Acid. Lowest member of dicarboxylic acid seres, COOH-COOH. Posonous, but not n small doses; occur in spinach, chocolate and rhubarb. The toxicity of rhubarb leaves is due to their high content of oxalic acid. Oxalic acid is normally excreted in human urine, 15-20mg per day, increased in diabetes and liver disease.

Oxidases. Enzymes that are able to oxidise compounds by removing hydrogen and adding from dehydrogenases, since the latter cannot pass the hydrogen directly on to oxygen but only to an intermediate.

Oxidation. Gain in oxygen, or loss of hydrogen or loss of electrons.

Oximetry. Refers to the continuous measurement of the amount of oxygen in the circulating blood.

Oxycalorimeter. Instrument which is used for measuring the oxygen used and carbon dioxide produced when a food is burred (as distinct from the bomb calorimeter, which measures the heat produced).

Oxyhaemoglobin. Refers to the form in which oxygen gets transported from the lungs to the tissues; a close combination of oxygen with the haemoglobi, which is readily decomposed.

Oxymyoglobin. Myoglobin is coloured protein in muscle which serves as a store of oxygen; it takes up oxygen to form oxymyoglobin, which is bright red, while myoglobin itself is purplishred. The surface of fresh meat which gets exposed to oxygen is bright red from the oxymyoglobin, while the interior of the meat is darker in colour where the myoglobin does not get not oxygenated.

Oxyntic Cells. Or parietal cells; glands in the stomach that produce hydrochloric acid of the gastric juice.

Oyster. Bivalve shellfish of the Ostrediae family, often eaten raw. Analysis per 100g of meat : 85g water, 11g protein, 1g fat, 50 kcal (220kj), 6mg Fe, 6-100 Zn, small amounts of most of the B vitamin group.

P

Palm Kernel Oil. Oil which is extracted from the kernel of the nut of Elaeis guineensis. The oil from the pulp is termed palm oil. Used for margarine and cooking fat.

Palm Oil. Oil extracted from the pericarp nor outer pulp beneath the outer skin of the nut from the oil palm, Elaeis guineensis. Coloured red due to high content of alpha-carotene (24mg per 100g) and beta-carotene (30mg) together with about 60mg tocopherols. Only 5-12% polyunsaturated fatty acids-linoleic acid. One of the major oils of commerce, and widely used in cooking fats and margarines.

Palm, Wild Date. Phoenix sylvestris, relative of the true date palm, P. dactylifera, grown in India as a source of sugar, obtained from the sap.

Panada. Refers to the mixture of fat, flour and liquid (such as stock or milk) mixed to a thick paste; used to bind mixtures such as chopped meat and also as the basis of souffles and chou pastry.

Panary Fermentation. Yeast fermentation of dough in bread-making.

Pancreas. Refers to a gland in the abdomen with two functions; it secretes (a) the hormone insulin, (b) the pancreatic juice. It is known by the butcher as sweetbread, or gut sweetbread, in distinction from chest sweetbread, which is thymus.

Pancreatic Juice. Digestive juice which gets produced by the pancreas and secreted into the duodenum; slightly alkaline, contains the enzymes trypsinogen, chymotrpsinoge, carboxypeptidase, aminopeptidase, lipase, amylase, maltase, sucrase, lactase and nucleases.

Pancreatin. Preparation obtained from the pancreas of animals and therefore containing the enzymes of pancreatic juice. Used as an aid to digestion.

Pancreozymin. An hormone which is produced by the intestinal mucosa which stimulates the pancreas to secrete enzymes.

Panettone. Italian, half bread-half cake.

Pangamic Acid. N- di-isopropyl derivative of glucuronic acid. It is a powerful methylating agent which is concerned with respiratory enzymes in cells. Also termed vitamin B , but no evidence that it is a dietary essential.

Pantothenic Acid. A vitamin having no numerical designation; chemically, beta-alanine plus pantoic acid. It is the part of the structure of coenzyme A, needed for the transfer of acetyl groups and therefore essential for the metabolism of fats and carbohydrates.

Dietary shortage never arises; universally distributed in all living cells, best sources being liver, kidney, yeast, bees royal jelly and fresh vegetables.

Deficiency symptoms is rats include greying of the hair, dermatitis, adrenal damage, in chicks, dermatitis, in dogs, gastrointestinal symptoms, but no definite pathological lesions in man. On the basis of the needs of animals, human requirements would be 6-8 mg per day. Also known as filtrate factor.

Pantoyltaurine. It is similar to pantothenic acid but with the carboxyl group replaced by a sulphonic acid group. It acts as an antagonist to the vitamin.

When given to man, gives rise to dizziness, postural hypotension, tachycardia, drowsiness and anorexia. Also called thiopanic acid.

Papain. Proteolytic enzyme from the juice of the papaya (Carica papaya) which is used in tenderising meat; sometimes called vegetable pepsin. Rate of reaction slow at room temperature, gets increased at 55-75°C maximum activity at 80°C And rapidly inactivated at temperatures higher than this; hence, the papain continues to tenderise the meat during the early stages of cooking.

Papaya. Pawpaw.

Papin's digester. Early version of the pressure cooker. Named after Papin, French physicist 1647-1712; originally invented for the purpose of softening bones for the preparation of gelatin.

Paraben. (methyl and propyl). Methyl and propyl parahydroxy benzoates. It finds used as preservatives at a concentration of 0.1%.

Parakeratosis. Disease of swine which is characterised by cessation of growth, erythema, seborrhoea and hyyperkeatosis of the skin; due to zinc deficiency, and essential fatty acids may be involved.

Parathyroid Glands. Four glands which are situated in the neck near to the thyroid gland but not connected with its function. They secrete the parathyroid hormone (parathormone) which controls the levels of the calcium in the blood and the excretion of phosphate in the urine.

Parboil. Partially cook. Of special interest in nutrition has been the parboiling of brown rice, that has been steaming of the rice in the husk before milling. The water-soluble B vitamins diffuse from the husk into the gain. When the rice is polished, the white rice contains far more of these vitamins than polished raw rice.

Parenteral Nutrition. Refers to the slow infusion of solution of nutrients into the veins through a cathether.

Parillin. Highly toxic gylcoside from sarsaparillia root; consists of glucose, rhamnose and parigenin. Also known as smilacin.

Parsely. Refers to the leaves of the herb Petroselium crispum or P. hertense, widely used as a garnish and flavouring. Rich in carotene and vitamin C but the amount consumed is too little to make a contribution to the diet. Turnip-rooted parsely is the root of

Petroselinum crispinum var tuberosum, also known as Hamburg parsely.

Parsnip. Root of Pastinaca sativa, eaten as a vegetable.

Parts per Million (ppm). Refers to a method of describing small concentrations and means exactly what the terms says. Mg per kg is also ppm. Usually used with regard to traces of metallic impurities and food additives, e.g., jam must not contain more that 40 ppm of sulphur dioxide.

Passion Fruit. Also called parchita, granadilla and water lemon; fruits of the tropical American vine, Passiflora species. Purple or greenish-yellow when ripe, watery pulp containing small seeds, used in fruit drinks.

Pasteurisation. Vegetative forms of many bacteria can be killed by mild heat treatment, pasteurisation, while total destruction of all bacteria and spores, sterilisation, requires higher temperatures for longer periods, often spoiling the product in the process. Pasteurisation will prolong the storage life of foods but usually only for a limited period.

Pasteurisation of milk is able to destroy all the pathogens, and although the milk will sour within a day or two, it is not a source of disease. Legally, pasteurisation of milk means maintaining at 145-150° F (63-66°C) for 30 minutes, followed by immediate cooling, or so-called 'high-temperature sort-time process', 161°F (72°C) for 15 seconds.

Pasteuriser. An equipment which is used to pasteurise liquids such as milk, fruit justice, etc. They function, in effect, as heat-ex-changers. The material to get pasteurised is passed continuously over heated plates, or through pipes, where it is heated to the required time, then immediately cooled.

Pathogens. Disease-causing bacteria. These are distinct from those that are harmless.

Patulin. Mycotoxin which is found in fruit juices from fruits infected with one of a variety of moulds (Penicillium expansum, Aspergillus calvatus, A. terreus and

Byssochlamys nivea). It is removed by fermentation and also pasteurisation.

Pavlov Pouch. A surgical technique which was introduced by Pavlov, in which a portion of the stomach is brought to the body wall. It is then possible to take a sample of the stomach contents directly from this pouch, as the secretion of the pouch is identical with that into the main part of the stomach.

Pawpaw (papaya). Large green or yellow melon-like fruit of the Carica papaya, a tree similar to the palm. It is the commonest tropical fruit second to the banana and is a rich source of vitamin A and C.

The proteolytic enzyme, papain, is obtained as the dried latex of the skin of the fruit by scratching it while still on the tree, and collecting the flow. In the tropics meat is often tendrised by wrapping in pawpap leaves.

PCM. Protein-calorie malnutrition.

Pea, Garden. Also called green pea; seed of the legume Pisum sativum. Widely available in frozen, dried and canned forms.

Pea, Processed. Garden Peas (Pisum sativum) that have matured on the plant and subsequently been canned.

Peanut Butter. Ground, roasted peanuts; commonly prepared from a mixture of Spanish and Virginia peanuts, as the first alone is too oily and the second is too dry. Separation of the oil is prevented by partial hydrogenation of the oil and the addition of emulsifiers.

Pear. Fruit of many species of Pyrus, cultivated varieties all descended from P. communis.

Pear, prickly. Fruit of the cactus opuntia, also called India fig, barberry fig, and tuna—an important part of the diet in certain areas of Mexico.

Peas. Seeds of a wide variety of leguminous plants including Cajanus (pigeon pea or red gram), Cicer arietinum (chick pea or Bengal gram), Pisum sativum (garden pea or green pea).

Pectase. An exzyme in the pith of citrus fruits which removed the methoxyl groups from pectin to form water-insoluble pectic acid. The intermediate compounds with varying numbers of methoxy groups are pectinic acids. It is also known as pectin esterase methly esterase and pectin methoxylase.

Pectinase. Enzyme present in the pith (albedo) cirtrus fruits, which gets hydrolysed pectins or pectic acids into smaller polygalacturonic acids, and finally galacturonic acid and its methyl ester.

Also known as pectolase and polygalacturonase.

Pectinesterase. Alternative name fore pectase.

Pectolasle. Alternative name for pectinase.

Pectosinase. Alternative name for protopectinase.

Pekar Test. Refers to a comparative test of flour colour. The flour gets pressed on a board with a smooth applicator and colour comparisons are made immersed in water.

Pelagic Fish. Refers to those that swim near the surface, compared with demersal fish, which live on the sea bottom. Pelagic fish are mostly of the oily type (herring, mackerel, pilchard), having up to 20% oil.

Pellagra. Disease which occurs due to deficiency of nicotinic acid. Symptoms include characteristic symmetrical dermatitis on exposed surfaces such as face and back of hands, mental disturbances and digestive disorders.

PEM. Protein-energy malnutrition.

Pemmican. Mixture of dried, powered meat and fat. Used as concentrated food source, e.g. on expeditions.

Penicillin. The first of the antibiotics which was isolated from the culture fluid of the mould Penicillium notatum, 1929. Active against a wide range of bacteria and of great value clinically. Not used as food preservative in case repeated small doses bring about penicillin resistance.

Penicillium. Moulds.

Pentosans. Complex carbohydrates which are widely distributed in plants e.g. fruit, wood cornocobs, oat hulls. These are not digested in the body but not down by acid to yield the 5- carbon sugars or pentoses.

Pentose. Simple sugar having 5 carbon atoms. The most

important has been ribose.

Pentosuria. Unexplained excretion of pentose sugars in the urine without any ill-effects. An inherited metabolic disorder almost wholly restricted to Ashkenazi (N. European) Jews.

P-enzyme. Potato phosphorylase which is specific for 1, 4-alpha links.

Pepper. Three types:

1. Sweet pepper, paprika, bell, pepper, bullnose pepper, Spanish name pimiento (not the same as pimento or allspice); fruits of the annual plant Capsicum annum. Red, yellow or brown fruits, often eaten law in salads when green and unripe; very variable size and shape; some varieties can be spicy but mostly non-pungent.
2. Red pepper, chilli (or chili), small red fruit of Capsicum frutescent, bushy, perennial plant. Usually sun-dried and therefore wrinkled, very pungent, ingredient of curry powder, pickles and tabasco sause. Cayenne pepper is made from the powdered dried fruits.
3. Black and white pepper, fruit of climbing vine, Piper nigru, grows in wet tropical conditions, fruits are peppercorns. Black pepper is made from sun-dried unripe pepper corns when red outer skin turns black. White papper is made by soaking ripe berries and rubbing off outer skin. Pungency due to alkaloids piperine, piperdine and chavicine.

Pepsi-cola. Trade name of a soft drink composed of sugar, vanilla, essential oils, spices and extract of coal nut coloured with caramel.

Pepsin. Proteolytic enzyme in the gastic juice which hydrolysis certain of the linkages of proteins to produce peptones. Functions only at acid pH, 1.5-2.5 secreted as the inactive precursor pepsinogen, which is activated by acid.

Peptides. Compounds formed when amino acids are linked together through the -CO-NH-linkage.

Peptones. Intermediate stage in the hydrolysis of proteins, distinguished from proteoses in not being precipitated by ammonium sulphate. The term is often used for any partial hydrolysate of proteins as , for example, 'bacteriological peptone' used as a medium for the growth of micro-organisms.

Peristalsis. A method of movement along the intestine, peristaltic waves, caused by contraction of a ring of muscle, preceded by a wave of relaxation.

Pernicious Anaemia. Refers to the form of anaemia which occurs due to a deficiency of vitamin B needed for maturation of the red blood cells. Almost always due to a defect in the absorption of vitamin B (termed the extrinsic factors), which needs the agency of factor produced in the gastric mucosa—the instrinsic factor—for absorption. Rarely due to a dietary shortage of vitamin B.

Peroxidase. A plant enzyme that is able to split hydrogen peroxide into water and oxygen, only when there is a substance present to accept the oxygen (unlike caralase, which splits peroxide into water and gaseous oxygen). Contains haematin in the molecule, and blood itself has a peroxidase—like activity that gets used in the benzidine test for blood.

Peroxide Number. Or peroxide value. Refers to measure of the oxidative rancidity of fats by determination of the peroxides present. It is measured by amount of iodine liberated from potassium iodide : peroxide value is the number milliliters of 0.002N sodium thiosulphate per gram of sample.

Perry. Fermented pear Juice, which is analogous to cider from apple.

Persian Berry. Yellow colour which is obtained from the berries of the buckthorn (Rhamnus) Family, legally permitted in food in most countries. Having the glucosides of two colouring matters, rhamnetin and rhamnazin.

Persimmon. Or date plum. Fruit of Diospyros kaki, Japanese persimmon. Which has the appearance of the tomato (called kaki in France), eaten raw, made into jams and jellies, and as persimmon pie made from the American persimmon (D). virginiana, in which the fruit is not cooked, since heating produces an acid taste.

Pervaporation. Evaporation from a colloidal suspension by heating in a collodion bag. If there are crystalloids present, they pass through the membrane and get deposited on the outside of the bag.

Petechiae. (petechial haemorrhages). Small, pin-point bleedings in the skin; one of the symptoms of scurvy.

Petit-grain Oils. Obtained from twigs and leaves of the bitter orange by steam distillation. These are similar to neroli oil but less fragrant.

Petit Pois. Small peas.

PGA. Pteroyl glutamic acid.

ph. Abbreviation of potential hydrogen. It is used to denote the degree of acidity of a substance. It is defined as the negative logarithm of the hydrogen-ion concentration in gram-atoms per litre. The scale runs from 0(1 gram of H ion per litre), extremely strongly acid, to 14 (one hundred-million-millionth of a gram of H ions) extremely strong alkaline.

Pure water is ph, 7 which is neutral; below 7 is acid, above is alkaline.

Phaeophytin. Formed from chlorophyll by the removal of the magnesium; occurs in acid medium. It is brownish-green in colour and accounts for the colour change when green vegetables are cooked.

Phagomania. Morbid obsession with food; also sitomania.

Phagophobia. Fear of food, also sitophobia.

Phase Inversion. Milk is an emulsion of fat in water, butter is an emulsion of water in fat. The change from cream to butter is called phase inversion.

Phaseolin. Globulin protein in kidney bean.

Phaseolunatin. Cyanogenetic glucoside found in certain legumes (such as lima bean, chick pea, common vetch), which gets hydrolysed to produce glucose, acetone and hydrocyanic acid; not proved harmful when present in the diet.

Phasin. Term originally used for the haemagglutinin from Phaseolus vulgaris but is now a term occasionally used for non-toxic plant agglutinins.

PHB Easter. p-Hydroxybezoic acid-ethyl and proyl esters and their sodium salts. Used as preservative in some countries.

Phenol Oxidases. Enzymes that are able to oxidise phenolic compounds to quinones. For example, monophenol oxidase in mushrooms; polyphenol oxidases in potato and apple are responsible for the development of the brown colour when the cut surface is exposed to air; tyrosinase in plants and animals which is responsible for brown and black pigmentation.

Phenylalanine. Refers to an essential amino acid. The non-essential tyrosine can partially replace phenylalanine in the diet.

Inability to metabolise phenylalanine has been an inherited diseases and causes mental disorder, phenylketonuria, which see.

Phenylketonuria. Inherited metabolic defect wherein the essential amino acid, phenylalanine, gets incompletely metabolised and the end-product, phenylpyruvic acid, gets excreted in the urine. The product affects the brain and causes imbecility. The effect can be moderated by strict limitation of the phenylalanine intake.

Phitosite. High-calorie food.

Phlorrhizin. Also spelled phioridzin and phlorhizin. A glycoside of plant origin; abolishes the renal threshold for glucose, which therefore appears in the urine (glycosuria). This is termed as renal diabetes or phlorhizig diabetes. Used to examine the formation of glucose from other ingredients of the diet.

Phosphate Bond, Energy-rich. Phosphates of organic compounds can be divided into two groups, depending on the amount of energy released when the phosphate portion get hydrolysed. (a) Lowenergy potential, the ordinary phosphates which liberate 1.22-1.5 kcal (e.g. phospho-sugars, phospho-glycerols, phosphoglyceric acids, phosphochorine); (b) high-energy potential or energy- rich phosphates, which liberate about 8-10 kcal (e.g. anhydrides, where phosphate is linked to phosphate, acidic enols such as phosphoenolypyruvic acid, acetyl phosphate and nitrogen linked to phosphate).

Phosphate-bond energy is the only form of energy that can be used by any living cell (muscular activity, osmotic work, the shock produced by the electric cell).

Adenosine triphosphate (ATP) is the key compound because it acts as a store of energy-rich phosphate bonds.

Phosphatides. Also called phospholipins or phospholipids. Fatty substances including phosphoric acid and a nitrogenous base in the molecule. Include lecithins, cephalins, sphingomyelins, and cerebrosides. Part of the structure of the brain and nervous tissue and involved in fat transport.

Also combined with proteins as lipoproteins.

Are party soluble in water as well as in fats and used in food technology as emulsifiers. From the dietary point of view they may be regarded as simple fats.

Phosphokinases. Enzymes that are able to transfer the phosphate radical, together with its energy, to or from adenosine di-or triphosphate. Various other molecules can be involved but one of the pair of reactants is adenosine di-or triphosphate.

Phospholipins. Phosphatides.

Phosphoprotems. Conjugated proteins having phosphate other than as nuclear acid (nucleoproteins) or lecithin (lipoproteins), e.g. casein from milk, ovovitellin from egg yolk.

Phosphoric Acid. May be one of three types—orthophosphoric acid (H_3PO_4), methaphosphoric acid (HPO_3) or pyrophosphoric acid ($H_4P_2O_7$). Used in acid—fruit flavored beverages such as lemonade.

Phosphorolysis. Refer to hydrolysis in which the elements of phosphoric acid get added at the broken linkage, e.g. the enzyme phosphorylase hydrolyses glycogen not to glucose but to glucose phosphate.

Phosphorus. This element is found in all biological tissues as phosphate, i.e., salts of phosphoric acid. In the body most of it (80%) occurs in the skeleton and teeth as calcium phosphate (Ca_3PO_4) about 10% in the musclers and 1% in the nervous system. It is of vital importance in metabolism, as many compounds (such as vitamin B_1 and B_2 glucose, adenosine, etc.) function as phopshates. The parathyroid glands control the level of phosphate in the blood.

Human dietary needs (about 1.3g per day) are always met; a deficiency never takes place in man. Phosphate deficiency, however, is one of the commonest deficiencies in livestock and gives rise to osteomalacia (also known as sweeny or creeping sickness).

Phosphate is also essential for plant growth.

Photosynthesis. The term used for the manufacture by plants of complex foods from water and carbon dioxide under the influence of sunlight.

Phrynoderma. Refers to a follicular hyperkeratosis of the skin (blocked pores or toad-skin) often encountered in malnourished people. Originally thought to be due to vitamin A deficiency but possible because of other deficiencies, and occurs mildy in well nourished people.

Physalin. Zeaxanthin dipalmitate; a caroteniod pigment which is found in the fruits of the Chinese lantern, Physalis.

Physin. Growth factor is needed by rats and occurring in liver; probably vitamin B.

Phytase. Phosphatase enzyme that hydrolyses phytin to inositol and phosphoric acid. Present in yeast, live, blood, malt and seeds. If a high level of yeast is used in baking with high-extraction flours, some of the phytin is broken down.

Phytic Acid. Inositol hexphosphoric acid. It is present in cereals, especially in the bran, fried legumes and some juts as both water-soluble salts (sodium and potassium) and insoluble salts of calcium and magnesium,

magnesium calcium phytate is phytin-approximately 12% calcium, 1.5% magnesium and 22% phosphorus. It is possibly involved in texture changes when potatoes and pulses are cooked (through binding of calcium). It can bind calcium, iron and zinc into insoluble complexes and it is not clear how far phytate reduces the availability of these minerals in the diet, especially because there are phytase enzymes in yeasts and legumes (and possibly in the human gut) which may liberate these minerals.

Phytoplankton. Minute plants which are floating in the sea which serve as the basic food for all marine life, since they photosynthesise.

Phytosterol. General name given to sterols which are occurring in plants. The chief of these is sitosterol (structurally closely related to cholesterol).

Pica. Perverted appetite (eating of earth, sand, clay, paper, etc.)

Piccalilli. Mixture of chopped, brine-preserved vegetables in mustard sauce (mustard and vinegar, thickened with tapioca starch, plus other spices, coloured with tartraxine).

Pickles, Dill. Pickles that have been fermented in a mixture of brine, cured dill weed, mixed spices and vinegar.

Pickling. Also called brining. Vegetables immersed in 5-10% brine undergo lactic acid fermentation, while the salt prevents the growth of undesirables. The sugars in the vegetables get broken down to lactic acid : at 25°C the process takes a few weeks, finishing at 1% acidity.

Pilchard. Fatty fish, sardina (clupea) pilchards; found in the sardine.

Pineapple. Fruit of the tropical plant Ananas sativus.

Pint, Reputed. 131/3 fluid oz.

Pipe. Cask for wine; volume varies with the type of wine, e.g. port, 115 gallons; Teneriffe, 100; Marsala, 93.

Pipecolic Acid. Chemically, it is piperidine-2-carboxylic acid. It is found in fresh green beans, potatoes and mushrooms, in fresh fruit and the dried seeds of legumes.

Its pharmacological effects are not known.

Pipis. Edible mollusc, Plebidonas deltoides, widely distributed around Australian coastline.

Pits. Stones from cherries, plum, peaches, apricots. The oil is extracted from these pits and find use in cosmetic, pharmaceuticals, conning sardines and as table oil. The press cake left behind contains the bitter principle, amygdalin.

Plankton. Minute organism, both plant (phytoplankton) and animal (zooplankton), drifting in the sea, which serve as the basic foodstuffs of marine life.

Plansifter. Refers to a nest of sieves which are mounted together so that material being sieved is divided into a number of fractions of different size. Widely used in flour milling.

Plantain. Variety of banana having higher starch and lower sugar content than desert bananas, picked when flesh is too hard to be eaten raw and used for cooking. Some varieties become sweet if left to ripen, others never develop a high sugar content.

Plasma, Blood. Blood consists of red cells, white cells and platelets, suspended in a clear protein solution, the plasma. Plasma proteins include fibrinogen, albumins and globulin. Of the 9% total plasma solids, 7% are proteins.

Plasmapheresis. Experimental method of reducing the serum proteins to a low level by removing part of the blood and returning only the red cells to the blood stream.

Plasma Proteins. In solution in the blood plasma-three main types, fibrinogen (0.2-0.4g per 100ml), albumin (4.4-5.3) and globulin (1.9-2.8).

Plate Count. In order to estimate the number of bacteria in a sample, it gets poured on to an agar plate, when each bacterial cell or group of cells multiplies to produce a colony which is visible to the naked eye. A count of number of colonies gives the number of bacteria in that portion of the sample that was taken.

Pasteurised milk contains about 100 000 bacteria per

millilitre; good-quality raw milk contains less than 500 000 per millilitre.

Pluck. Butchers' term for heart, liver and lungs of an animal.

Plum. Numerous species of Prunus.

Analysis per 100g : 60 kcal (0.24 MJ), 100g carotene, 0.5gm nicotinic acid, 5mg vitamin C.

Pneumatic conveying. Refers to the transfer of material in powder form by means of air currents. Applied to flour, sugar, cement, etc.

Pneumatic Dryers. The material gets dried almost instantaneously in a turbulent stream of hot air, which also acts as a conveyor system. It is applicable to powdered, granular and flaky materials.

Pneumatic Ring Dryer. Refers to a pneumatic dryer in which the product travels several times through a ring duct, impelled by hot air, and the drying time, temperature and rate of flow of the material can be controlled. It is used for starch, mashed potatoes, cereals flour, powdered soups.

Poach. To cook for a short time in a shallow layer of liquid kept at a temperature just below the boiling point.

POEMS. Polyoxyethylene monostearate.

Poikilotherms. Cold-blooded animals, those whose temperature gets varied with their environment.

Polarised Light. Ordinary light vibrates in many planes; after passing through a crystal of quartz of 'polaroid', it vibrates in only one plane, i.e. it gets polarised. Many naturally occurring compounds in solution are having the ability to rotate the plane of polarised light, i.e. they are optically active.

Polarograph. Instrument which is used to measure traces of metallic ions by change in electric current. The test solution is the electrolyte between two mercury electrodes; a continuously increasing negative potential is applied to the cathode and the change in current with voltage is recorded-the polarogram. The rise in current at a particular voltage gives rise to a measure of the concentration of the metal ion present.

Polished Rice. Rice.

Polycythaemia. Refers to the increase in the number of red blood cells. It results from strenuous physical exercise, residence at high altitudes, administration of drugs or cobalt, and certain diseases.

Polydextrose, Modified. Randomly bonded glucose polymer which is prepared by heating glucose and sorbitol with citric acid; because of the random bonding and occasional diester linkage, it is more resistant to enzymic digestion than normal polymers and 60% gets excreted in faeces undigested-so providing only about 1 kcal/g; hence, termed non-sweetening sucrose replacement, or bulking agent.

Polymorphism. Refers to the ability to crystallise in two more different firms. For example, depending on the conditions under which it gets solidified, the fat tristearin can form three kinds or crystals, each of which has a different melting point, namely, 54 65 and 71°C.

Polymyxin. Antibiotic which is isolated from Bacillus polymyxin (Bacillus aerosporin). There are several polymyxins, of which polymyxin. A is aerosporin. They are polypeptides, active against coliform bacteria; apart from clinical use, they are of value of controlling infection in brewing.

Polyols. Sugar alcohols like glycerol, sorbitol, inositol, etc.

Polyose. Polysaccharide.

Polyoxyethylene. Monoglycerides are soluble in fat, but by reacting with eathylene oxide the resulting polyoxyethylene derivatives become water-soluble to whatever degree is needed. These compounds a e polyoxyethylene ester, ethers, sorbitol esters etc. They are valuable as emulsifying agents in bakery.

One of the best-known has been polyoxythelene stearate which is used as a crumb-softener.

Polyphagia. Excessive or continuous eating.

Olyphosphates. Complex phosphates which are added to foods, in particular meat products; they prevent sausage discoloration, aid mixing of the fat, speed penetration of the brine in curing, bring about protein fibres of meat to retain more water and swell (so improving texture).

Polysaccharides. Complex carbohydrates which are formed by the condensation of large numbers of monosaccharide units e.g. starch, glycogen, cellulose, dextrins, insulin. On hydrolysis the simple sugar gets liberated.

Polysaccharose. Polysaccharide.

Pomace. Residue of crushed apple pulp after expressing juice. This term is also applied to any pressed fruit pulp and to fish from which oil has been expressed.

Pombe. African beer prepared from millet seed.

Pomegranate. Punica granatum. Juice contained in a pulpy sac which is surrounding each of a mass of seeds—outer skins contains tannin and therefore bitter. Sweet juice used to prepare grenadine syrup for alcoholic and fruit drinks.

Pomelo. Also spelled 'Pomeloe' and 'Pummelo'; alternative name shaddock; Citrus grandis, from which the grapefruit gets decended.

Pomes. Botanical name for fruit which is formed by the enlargement of the receptacle which becomes fleshy and surrounds the carpels, e.g. apple, pear.

Ponderal Index. Refers to an index of adipose tissue; height divided by the cube root of the body weight; high for thin people, low for fat people.

Ponderocrescive. Foods tending to increase weight : easily gaining weight; opposite to pondoperditive - stimulating weight loss.

Poonac. Refers to the residue of coconut after the extraction of the oil.

Popcorn. Variety of maize, Zea mays, that expands on heating.

Pork Carcass. Analysis, fat, per 100g : protein 8.8g, fat 49g, kcal 480 (2.0MJ), Fe 11mg, carotene nil, vitamin B_1 0.31mg, vitamin C nil.

Porphyra. Red alga which is cultivated in Japan to make

'Komba' In some countries it is collected from these to make laver bread.

Porphyria. Refers to clinical disorder of metabolic pathway of haem synthesis in which porphyrins get excreted in the urine and faeces, and, in so me disorders, deposited in the skin.

Porphyrins. Compounds consisting of a ring system of four pyrrole nuclei joined by the = CH-bridges. Chlorophyll is a magnesium porphyrin; haem is an iron porphyrin.

Porphyrospsin. Refers to the photosensitive pigment in the retinas of the eyes of fresh-water fish, having dehydro retinol-anaogouss to rhodopsin in the eyes of marine fish, mammals, birds and amphibians.

Port Wine. Fortified wine, 16% alcohol, 12% sugars, 160 kcal (660KJ) per 100 ml. Designated 'ruby' (the youngest and seetest), 'tawny' (aged in the wood) and 'vintge' (aged in the bottle).

Posset. A drink which is made of hot milk curdled with ale or wine, sometimes thickened with bread crumbs and spiced. Formerly used as remedy for colds.

Potassium. An element which is widespread in nature and present in the human body in amounts of about 250g. Mostly present inside the cells. One of the most important of the plant nutrients.

Potassium Nitrate. Nitrates, nitrites, slatpetre.

Potassium Sorbate. Sorbic acid.

Potato Flour. Dried potato tuber.

Analysis per 1 (0g : starch 73g protein 8 5g, fat 0.4g, kcal 349 (1.47MJ), Ca 30mg, Fe 3mg, vitamin A nil, vitamin B_1 0.21mg, vitamin B_2 0.1mg, nicotinic acid 5mg, vitamin C 20mg.

Potato Starch. Also called farina. It is prepared from potato tuber and widely used as a stabilising agent when gelatinised. Large grains gelatinise very easily when heated.

Potato, Sweet. Tubers of herbaceous climbing plant Ipomoea batatas. The flesh may be white, yellow or pink (if carotene is present); the leaves are edible.

Analysis per 100g : starch 22g protein 1.1g, fat 0.3g, kcal 97(0.41MJ), Fe 0.mg, carotene 150ug, vitamin $B_1$0.08mg, vitamin $B_2$0.04mg, nicotinic acid 0.5mg, vitamin C 19mg.

Pot-au-feu. Traditional French dish which is made by stewing meat with vegetables. Soup is made from the liquor.

Pottle. English wine measure of half a gallon.

Pound Cake. Rick cake having a pound, or equal quantities, of each of the major ingredients.

PPM. Parts per million

Praline.

1. A paste of nuts and sugar which is used on cakes or as a chocolate fulling.
2. Refers to a sugar-coated almond.

Prawns. Refer to the shellfish of various tribes of suborder Macrura. Large fish of species of Palaemondiae, Penaeidae and Pandalidae are prawns, smaller fish are shrimps.

In addition, deepwater prawn is Pandalus borealis, common pink shrimp is Pandalous montagui, brown shrimp is species of Crangon.

PRE. Protein retention efficiency.

Precursor, Enzyme. Some enzymes get secreted as an inactive precursor that has to undergo a reaction before it shows normal activity. Thus, trypsin is secreted as inactive trypsinoge, which must reach with enterokinase before it becomes active, similarly pepsinogen and chymotrypsinogen.

Premier Jus. Best-quality suet which is prepared from oxen and sheep kidneys. The fat is chilled, shredded and heated at moderate temperature. When pressed, premier jus, like rendered tallow, separates into a liquid fraction (oleo oil or liquid oleo) and a solid fraction (oleostearin or solid tallow).

Preservation. Refers to the protection of food from deterioration by micro-organisms, enzymes and oxidation-by cooling, destroying the micro-organisms and enzymes by heat treatment, or irradiation, reducing their activity through dehydration or the addition of chemical preservatives, and by smoking, salting and pickling.

Preservatives. Substances which are capable of retarding or arresting the deterioration of food; examples are sulphur dioxide, benzoic acid, specified antibiotics, salt, acids and essential oils.

Pretzels. Hard brittle German biscuits made from flour, water, shortening, yeast and salt.

Proenzymes. Inactive precursors to enzymes, also termed as zymogens.

Proenzymes. Inactive precursors to enzymes, also termed as zymogens.

Profiteroles. Refer to the small rounds of chou pastry which are used as a garnish for clear soups or consommes; or filled with cream, baked and sweetened with syrup and chocolate sauce.

Progoitrin. Substances occurring in plant foods which get converted into goitrins, e.g., glucoside of hydroxybutenyl isothiocyanate.

Prolamins. Refers to proteins which are insoluble in 70-80% alcohol; e.g., wheat gliadin, corn zein, barley hordein, malt bynin. They are low in lysine, rich in proline and glutamic acid.

Proline. Refers to anon-essential amino acid. Chemically, pyrrolidine carboxylic acid.

Proof Spirit. Refers to a method of describing the alcohol content of spirits. Proof spirit is having 57.07% alcohol by volume and 49.24% by weight in many countries such as U.K. in the USA it contains 50% alcohol by volume. Spirits are described as under or over proof. A mixture 30 degrees over proof contains in 100 volumes as much alcohol as 130 volumes of proof spirit : 30 degrees under proof means that 100 volumes contain as much alcohol as 70 volumes of proof spirit. In Germany percentage alcohol by weight is used, in Italy and France it is percentage by volume.

Proof spirit is a solution of alcohol of such strength that

it will ignite when mixed with gunpowder; specifically, at 10°C it weight 12/13 parts of an equal volume of distilled water.

Propionates. Refers to the salts of propionic acid, CH_3CH_2COOH. The free acid and its sodium and calcium salts find use as mould inhibitors, e.g., on cheese surfaces; also to inhibit rope in bread.

Propionic acid gets formed in the rumen of cattle together with acetic and butyric acids, and all three are converted into milk constituents.

In the body it gets metabolised to pyruvic acid, which is normally formed in body, and thus considered harmless.

Protamines. The simplest natural proteins, having only a limited number of amino acids, chiefly the basic ones, especially arginine. Soluble in water; not coagulated by heat; so basic that they form salts with strong mineral acids, e.g. salmine from salmon sperm, sturine from sturgeon sperm, clupeine from herring sperm, scombrine from mackerel sperm.

Proteans. Slightly altered proteins, probably an early stage of denaturations, which have become insoluble.

Protein, Bence-jones. Unusual protein excreted in the urine in multiple myelomatosis, leukaemia and eczema; coagulates at 55°C and redissolves on boiling.

Protein, Crude. Total nitrogen multiplied by 6.25.

Protein Efficiency Ratio. Refers to a measure of the nutritive value of proteins carried out on young growing animals. It is defined as the gain in weight per gram of protein eaten. The maximum values, e.g. egg protein, are about 4.4. Zero values are obtained for those proteins which, when fed alone, do not permit growth, but may still have some limited value.

Protein-energy Malnutrition. Refers to a marked dietary deficiency of both energy and protein which includes as spectrum of disorders ranging from kwashiorkor to marasmus; the major cause of deaths among infants in developing countries.

Protein-energy Ratio. Protein content of a food or diet

which is expressed as ratio between energy from protein and total energy. Previously termed protein calories per cent, being expressed as a percentage of total calories supplied by protein.

Protein Equivalent. Refers to a measure of the digestible nitrogen of an animal feedingstuff in terms of protein. It can be measured by direct feeding or calculated from the digestible pure protein plus half the digestible non-protein nitrogen.

Protein, First Class. First and second class proteins are obsolete terms indicating those of high or low nutritive value, generally, but not invariably, animal and plant protein, respectively.

Protein Milk. Partially skimmed lactic acid milk plus milk curd (prepared from whole milk by rennet precipitation). It is richer in protein and poorer in fat than ordinary milk-supposed to be better tolerated in digestive disorders. Also called albumin milk and eiweiss milch.

Protein Quality. Refers to the measure of the usefulness of a protein food for various purposes, including growth, maintenance, repair of tissue, formation of new tissue and, in animals, production of eggs, wool and milk. Various methods of measurements are used to serve as an index of quality.

Proteins. Essential constituents of all living cells. They are distinguished from fats and carbohydrates in containing nitrogen; basically composed of carbon, hydrogen, oxygen, nitrogen, sulphur and sometimes phosphours. All proteins are composed of large combinations of 20 amino acids (some bacterial proteins certain additional unusual amino acids). Meat, fish, eggs, cheese, hair, leather, fur, and many hormones are having a high protein content.

Proteins, Conjugated. The molecule is having protein and a non-protein prosthetic group; e.g., nucleoproteins, glycoproteins phosphorproteins, chromoproteins, lipoproteins.

Protein Score. Refers to chemical method of defining the nutritional value of proteins; the ratio of the amount of the limiting essential amino acid in the protein, to the target value.

Protein Shift. Name applied in flour milling to the phenomenon in which the protein content of the smaller particles of flour (up to 15 microns) has been higher, namely 15-20% than that of the flour as a whole, 8-14%, while particles of intermediate size, 15-35 microns have a lower proteins content than the flour as a whole.

Proteolysis. Refers to the partial degradation products of proteins; soluble in water. The stage of breakdown are protein- proteoses-peptones-polypeptides-amino acids. The proteoses are distinguished from peptones in that they are precipitated from solution by ammonium sulphate, whereas peptones are not.

Primary proteoses get precipitated with half-saturated ammonium sulphate; secondary proteoses require full saturation.

Prothrombin. Protein of the plasma which is involved in coagulation of the blood.

Protopectinase: Refers to the enzyme in the pith of citrus fruits which converts protopectin into pectin with the resultant separation of the plants cells from one another. Also called pectosinase and pectosase.

Proving. In bread-making in fermentation of the dough at the stage just before it goes into the oven.

Provitamin. Refers to a substance that get converted into a vitamin, such as 7-dehydrocholesterol, which is converted into vitamin D. In the old nomenclature carotene was called provitamin A.

Proximate Analysis. Nearly complete analysis which is comprising protein, fat and, ash, and by subtracting these from the total, calculating 'carbohydrate by difference '. The last value can be corrected for crude fibre.

Pseudoglobulin. Water-soluble globulin which does not get precipitated from salt solutions by dialysis against distilled water. Pseudo-globulin fractions are found in blood serum, in animal tissues, and in milk.

P.S Ration. Refers to the ratio between polyunsaturated and saturated fatty acids. Low ratio believed to be a risk factor in atherosclerosis and coronary heart disease. Ratio in western diets about 0.6; suggested that risk reduced if that ratio is changed towards 1.0.

Psychrophillic Bacteria. Prefer temperatures 15-20°C (59-68°F) and will still grow at and below 0°C (32°F)—that is, in cold stores. Bacteria of the genera Achromobacter, Flavobacterium, pseudomonas and Micrococcus; Torulopsis yeasts; and moulds of the genera Penicillium, Cladosporium, Mucor and Thamnidium can all develop at low temperatures.

Temperatures must be reduced to about-10° (13°F) before growth stops, but the organisms are not killed and will regrow when the temperature rises.

Psyllium. Also called plantago or flea seed-Plantago psyllium. Small, dark reddish-brown seeds which form a mucilaginous mass with water, taken medicinally to assist the passage of intestinal contents.

Ptomaines. Loosely used name for amino compounds which are formed by decarboxylation of amino acids during putrefaction of animal proteins-putrescine from arginine, cadaverine from lysine, muscarine in mushrooms, neurine formed by dehydration of choline.

Ptyalin. Old name for salivary amylase.

Pudding, Black. Also called blood pudding. Traditional European dish made with sheep or pig blood and suet, originally together with oatmeal, liver and herbs stuffed into membrane casings shaped like a horseshoe.

Pudding, Hasty. Old dish which is made from oatmeal boiled with water for only 2-3 minuets; the finished dish is very low in water content.

Puff Pastry. During preparation continuous layers of fat get formed between layers of dough; upon baking steam accumulates between the dough layers and makes them to expand, forming large spaces between thin layers of pastry.

Pulque. Sourich beer which is produced by the rapid natural fermentation of aquamiel, the sweet mucilaginous sap of the agave. Contains 6% alcohol by volume, common in Central and South America.

Pulses. Name which is given to the dried seeds (matured on the plant) of legumes such as peas, beans and lentils. In the fresh, wet form they are having about 90% water, but the dried form is having about 10% water and can be stored.

Pumpernicked. Heavy, black bread made from rye originating from Germany. Name derived from Napoleon's remark that it was 'pain pour Nicole' (this horse).

Purothionine. Lipoprotein in wheat having fungicidal properties. May be the factor known to bakers and brewers and 'yeast poison': similar compound found in barley is called hordothionine. Used to classify yeasts.

Putrescine. Tetramethylene-diamine. It is formed by decarboxylation of arginine.

Pyrexia. Rise in body temperature.

Pyrithiamine. Pyridine analogue of thiamin. It is the antagonistic to the vitamin.

Pyrogens. Substances which are produced by living bacteria (not yeasts or moulds). They cause a rise in body temperature on injection. Thus any material that has been infected may, despite subsequent sterilisation, have pyrogens and be unsuitable for injection. Pyrogens are not destroyed by heat and water supplies can be pyrogenic.

Pyruvic Acid. $CH_3COCOOH$. Occupies a central position in the metabolism of carbohydrate. The anaerobic breakdown of glucose produces pyruvic acid, which then gets oxidised via the tricarboxylic and cycle to carbon dioxide and water.

Q

Q-enzyme. A factor which is isolated from potatoes that catalyses the formation of branching linkages of the 1, 6-alpha type in starches; the reaction appears to be irreversible, i.e. the Q-enzyme cannot hydrolyse these 1, 6-alpha linkages.

Quart, Reputed. Customary measure in relation to bottled wine and spirits is a 'bottle' known as a reputed quart, approximately two-third of an imperial quart, or 26 fluid ounces. Reputed pints is 13 fluid ounces.

Quebracho. Or aspidosperma. It is obtained from the bark of Aspidosperma quebracholbanco ; used as source of tannins and alkaloids.

Queen Substance. Refers to the material secreted by the queen bee which inhibits the ovaries of the worker bees and stops them constructing queen cells. Thought to be chemically 10-hydroxy delta-2-decenoic acid.

Quenelle. Refers to a ball of chopped spiced meat or fish.

Quercetin. Refers to a flavone found in onion skins, tea, hops, horse chest nuts; the disaccharide derivative having rhamnose and glucose in routine.

Quetelet's Index. Index of adiposity; weight (kg) divided by square of height (metres); 25 considered 'normal'.

Quick Breads. Term for baked goods like bisuits, muffins, popovers, griddles, cakes, waffles and dumplings, in which no yeast is used, but the raising carried out quickly with baking powder or other chemical agents.

Quick Freezing. A rapid freezing of food by exposure to a blast of air at a very low temperature. Unlike slow freezing, small crystals of ice get formed which do not rupture the cells of the food and so the structure is relatively undamaged. A quick frozen food is commonly defined as one that has been cooled from a temperature of 0 C to 5 C or lower, in a period of not more than 2 hours and then cooled to-18 C.

Quillaja. Or soapbark; the dried bark of quillaja saponaria, which is having sapotoxin, tannin and quillaja. Used to produce foam in soft drinks and shampoos and fire extinguishers.

Quince. Pear-shaped sour fruit of Cydonir species, with flesh similar to that of the apple. It is rich in pectin and used chiefly in jams and jellies; used to be known as the apple and the vine.

Analysis per 100g : water 83 g, protein 0.4g, fat trace, carbohydrate 6g, kcal 25(0.1MJ), vitamin C 15mg.

R

Remekin.

1. Porcelain or earthenware mould in which mixture gets baked and then brought to the table. Paper souffle cases nowadays called ramekin cases.

2. Formerly the name given to toasted cheese: now tarts filled with cream cheese are called ramekins.

Randomisation. As used of fats, is the same as interesterification.

Rape. Brassica napus. It is closely related to garden swede. Also known as cole or clossed. Seed used as source of edible oil, although its content of erucic acid has raised problems. Residual oilcake used for animal feed, although it is having goitrigens.

Raspberry. Fruit of Rubus idaeus.

Rastrello. Sharp-edged spoon which is used to cut out the pulp from halved orange or others citrus fruit.

Ratafia. Flavouring essence which is made from bitter almonds; also a small light macaroon biscuit used in trifles; also a liqueur made from plum, peach and apricot kernels and bitter almonds.

Ravioli. Square envelope of pasta which is stuffed with minced meat.

Raw Sugar. Brown unrefined sugar, 96-98% pure. Contaminated with mould spores, bacteria, cane firbe, and dirt.

RDA. Recommended daily (or dietary) allowance or amount

(of energy and nutrients).

RDI. Recommended daily intake or recommended dietary intake (or energy and nutrients).

Reciprocal Ponderal Index. Height divided by cube root of weight; index of adiposity.

Recknagel's Phenomenon. Refers to the slight rise in specific gravity of milk which many continute for up to 12 hours after milking; total effect may be equivalent to 0.15% solids not fat in the milk. The cause has not been explained.

Recommended Intakes (of nutrients). Daily amount of each nutrient and of energy recommended as being adequate to maintain health. These are based on measured requirements plus a calculated surplus to take care of individual variation (except for energy which is based on observed average intakes).

Rectifying Column. Refers to a distillation column which is so arranged that the vapour condenses and redistils many times before it is finally condensed to form the distillate and so is purified to a greater degree than in simple distillation.

Red Colours. Red 10B- disodium salt of 8-amino-2phenylazo-1-naphthol-3,6 -disulphonic acid.
Red 2G disodium salt of 8-acetamido-2- phenylazo-1-naphthol-3,6-disulphonic acid.
Red FB- disodium salt of 2- (4-(1-hydroxy-4-sulpho-2-naph-thylazo)-3-sulphopheny1)-6-sulphonic acid.

Red Herrings. Herrings which are well salted and smoked for about 10 days. Bloaters are salted less and smoked for a shorter time; kippers light salted and smoked overnight.

Reducing Sugars. Sugars that are having the aldehydic or ketonic reducing group e.g. glucose, fructose, lactose, pentoses. They are tasted for by their ability to reduce reagents like Fehling's, Benedict's.

Reduction. Loss of oxygen, or gain in hydrogen or gain of electrons.

Reductones. Enediols which may get formed from sugars

carrying a free carboxyl group by heating in alkaline solution. The simplest is hydroxyglycolaldehyde. Reductones may be formed in carbohydrate foods during heat processing and as they have similar proper ties to vitamin C they interfere with its estimation.

Similar interferring substances are reductinic acids formed by acid treatment of pentoses.

Reference Man. Refers to an arbitrary physiological standard. It may be defined as a man of 25 years, healthy, weight 65kg, living in a temperate zone of a mean annual temperature of 10, assumed to require an average daily intake of 3200 kcal (135MJ).

Reference Protein. Refers to a theoretical concept of the perfect protein which finds use with 100% efficiency at whatever level it is fed in the diet. Used as means of expressing recommended intakes.

The nearest approach to this theoretical protein are egg and human milk proteins, which are used with 90-100% efficiency when fed at low levels in the diet (4%) but not when fed at high levels (10-15%).

Reference Woman. Refers to an arbitrary physiological standard. It may be defined as a woman of 25 years, weight 55kg, engaged in general household duties or light industry, using 2300 kcal (9.7MJ) per day, and as reference man, living in a temperate zone at a mean annual temperature of 10°C.

Refractive Index. Refers to a measure of the bending or refraction of a beam of light on entering a denser medium : the ratio between the sine of the angle of incidence of the ray of light and sine of the angle of refraction. It has been constant for pure substances under standard conditions. Used as a measure of sugar or total solids in solution in, purity of oils, etc.

Refractometer. Opical instrument which is used to measure the refractive index, which see.

The Abbe refractometer has two prisms between which is spread the substance under examination (jam, fruit, juice, sugar syrup, etc.) and light gets reflected through the solution. The immersion refractometer dips into the solution.

Refrigeration. Preservation; psychrophilic bacteria.

Rehfuss Tube. Instrument which is used for removing samples of food from the stomach after a test meal. It is a small-diameter tube with a slotted metal tip. Another type is the Ryle tube, which see.

Reichert-Meissl Value. Refers to a measure of the volatile fatty acids in fats. Defined as m of N/10 NaOH required to neutralise the distillate from 5g of fat, = Reichert-Meissl number.

Relative Humidity. Refers to the method of expressing moisture content of the atmosphere (relative to saturation at the same temperature). Spoilage organisms can grow and sporce can germinate only at particular moisture levels so long as the moisture is 'available'. The high sugar content of jam, for example, makes water unavailable so that although the food is high in water content, organisms cannot grow, available water is signified by a_w.

Release Agents. Substances which are applied to tinned or enameled surfaces of plastics to prevent the food adhering, e.g., fatty acid amides, microcrystalline waxes, petrolatums, starch, methyl cellulose.

Renal Threshold. Refers to the blood level of a particular substance at which it gets excreted through the kidney. For example, renal threshold of glucose is about 180mg per 100 m, and diabetics excrete glucose because this level is exceeded. Various drugs can reduce the renal threshold.

Rendering. Refers to the process of liberating the fat form. The fat cells that constitute the adipose tissue. Dry rendering, heating the fat dry, or wet rendering, when water is present.

Rennet. Extract of calf stomach. It is having the enzyme rennin which clots milk. Used in cheese-making and for junkets.

Rennet, Vegetable. Name given to proteolytic enzymes

which are derived from plants, such as bromelain (from the pineapple) and ficin (from the fig).

Rennin. Enzyme in the abomasum of calves and the stomach of human infants which clots milk by precipitation of the casein. No evidence that it plays any part in digestion in the adult.

Rentschlerising. Sterilising by treatment with ultraviolet light. It was named after Dr. H.C Rentschler, who developed the lamp.

R-enzyme. An enzyme which is present in beans and potatoes that splits the 1,6 glucosidase found in muscle. Also known as the 'debranching' factor.

Resazurin Test. Methylene blue test.

Respiratory Quotient. Refers to the ratio between the volume of carbon dioxide produced when a substance is oxidised, and the volume of oxygen used. In respiration in man the oxidation of carbohydrate causes RQ of 1.0; of fat, 0.71; and of protein, 0.8.

Restoration. With reference to food, usually implies the addition of nutrients to replace those lost in processing, as in milling of creals.

Reticulin. Refers to one of the structural elements (together with elastin and collagen) of skeletal muscle. Chemically it is identical with collagen but histologically it stains black with silver, while collagen stains yellow or brown; it is thought to be a precursor or a degraded form of collagen.

Reticulocyte. Young form of the red blood cell (normocyte or erythrocyte) in which the remains of the nucleus has been visible as a reticulum very few are seen in the normal blood; they get retained in the marrow until mature; but on remission of anaemia, when there is a high rate of production, reticulocytes appear in the blood stream (reticulocytosis).

Reticulo-endothelial System. A 'system' of cell distributed throughout the body, with phagocytic properties. Present in spleen, bone marrow, live, and lymph nodes, and are also mobile in the tissues and blood stream. They act as scavengers of tissue debris and bacteria.

The reticulo-endothelial system also removes red blood cells when they have completed their life of 120 days. The iron is recovered for further use, and the rest of the haemoglobin is converted to bile pigments in the faeces and urobilin in the urine.

Retinal. Aldhyde of retinol. It was formerly termed vitamin A aldehyde.

Retinoic Acid. An acid which is derived from retinol, formerly vitamin A acid.

Retinol. Formerly termed vitamin A alcohol.

Retort. In connection with food technology, an autoclave.

Retrogradation. Refers to a change in gelatinised starch occurring on storage which causes reduced solubility and a change of texture. It is important in products like dehydrated potatoes and baked products.

Rhamnose. A methyl pentose sugar; 33% sweetness of sucrose.

Rheology. Refers to the science of deformation and flow of matter. In food technology it involves brittleness and plasticity of fast, soughs, milk curds, grains, etc.

Rhiotin. Unidentified urinary excretion product of biotin, together with motin and triotin.

Rhodamine B. Refers to the hydrochloride of diethyl-m-amino phenol phthalein—until recently used as a red colour in mint paste and mint rock but now permitted in most other countries.

Rhodopsin. Visual purple; vitamin A.

Rhubarb. Refers to leaf-stalks of perennial plant. Rheum rhaponticum. Having only traces of protein and carbohydrate. High con tent of oxalate; leaves are toxic for this reason.

Riboflavin. Vitamin B_2.

Ribose. The pentose sugar of outstanding physiological importance; it is part of vitamin B_2, of coenzyme I and II, of adenylic acid, and in the nucleoproteins either as ribose or desoxyribose.

Ribosomes. Particles which are found in animal cells,

plants, yeasts, and as a major constituent of bacterial cytoplasm—believed to be the site of protein synthesis; composed of ribonucleic acid.

Rice. Grain of oryza sativa; major food in many countries. Rice when threshed is called paddy, and is covered with a fibrous husk comprising nearly 40% of the grain. When the husk has been removed, brown rice is left. When the outer bran layers up to the endosperm and germ are removed, the ordinary white rice of commerce of polished rice is obtained (usually polished with glucose and talc). In conversion to polished rice there occurs considerable loss of vitamin B_1 (and nicotinic acid); hence the widespread occurrence of berriberri among rice-eating peoples.

Rice, Glutinous. For most purposes separate rice grains are wanted that do not stick together in a glutinous mass. Glutinous rice is rich in soluble starch, dextrin and maltose and on boiling the grains adhere in a sticky mass; this rice for use for sweetmeats and cakes.

Rice, Hungry. Refers to a variety of millet, Digitaria exilis. It is important in West Africa.

Rice Paper. Refers to smooth white paper which is made from the pith of a tree peculiar to Formosa. It is edible, and macaroons and similar biscuits are baked on it and the paper can be eaten with biscuits.

Rice Parboiled. Rice that has been partially cooked before milling, so that some of the water-soluble B vitamins migrate into the grain and less gets lost when the rice is subsequently milled to white rice.

Rice Red. West African species, Oryza glaberrima, with red bran layer.

Rice, Unpolished. Rice which is undermilled in that the husk, germ and bran layers have been partially removed.

Rice, Wild. Also known as zizanie. Tuscarora rice, Indian rice and American wild rice; Zizania aquatica. Native to E. North America, grows 12 feet high; long, thin greenish grain; little is grown and difficult to harvest, so is strictly a gourmet food. Higher in protein content than ordinary rice at 14%, fat 0.7%, carbohydrate 74%, fibre 1.5%.

Ricing. Culinary term which means cutting into small pieces about the size of rice grains.

Pickets. Malformation of the bone in growing children due to shortage of vitamin C leading to poor absorption of calcium. In adults the equivalent is osteomalacia.

Rickets, Refractory. Rickets that does not respond to normal doses of vitamin D but needs massive doses; it is suggested that refractory rickets is a congential abnormality.

Riffle Flumes. Washing equipment which is consisting of stepped channels along which the product being washed is carried in a flow of water; stones and grit are retained on the steps.

Rigor Mortis. Stiffening of muscle that occurs after death. As the flow of blood ceases, anaerobic metabolism gives rise to the formation of lactic acid and the soft, pliable muscle becomes stiff and rigid. If meat is hung in a cool place for few days (i.e. 'conditioned'), the meat softens again. Fish similarly undergo rigor morits but is generally of shorter duration than in mammals.

Ringer's solution. Solution of the chlorides of sodium, potassium and calcium in which isolated tissues will continue to survive (960 ml of 0.154M NaCl, 20ml 0.154MCaCl^2.)

Roast. Originally this term was meant to cook meat over an open fire on a spit; now refers to cooking in an enclosed oven, and so is 'dryheating'. With meat the juices get squeezed out and evaporate on the surface, producing the Maillard complex characteristic of roasted meat.

Robison Easter. Name given to a mixture of glucose-6-phosphate and fructose-1 phosphate, which are intermediary stages in glucose metabolism.

Rocambole. Allium scordoprasum. A mild variety of garlic, also called sand leek.

Rochelle Salt. Potassium sodium tartrate. It is used to combine with the copper in Fehling's test for reducing sugars.

Roe. Hard roe is the egg of the female fish; soft roe is from the male fish, also known as milt.

Roller Dryer. The material to the dried has been spread over the surface of internally heated rollers and drying has been complete in a few seconds. The rollers rotate against a knife that scrapes off the dried film as soon as it forms.

Roller Mill. Pairs of horizontal cylindrical rollers which are separated by only a small gap and revolving at different speeds.

The material is thus ground and crushed in the one operation. Used in flour milling.

Roll-on Closure (RO). Aluminium or lacquered tinplate cap for sealing on to narrow-necked bottles having a threaded neck. The unthreaded cap is moulded on to the neck of the bottle and forms as air-tight seal.

Root Beer. Non-alcoholic carbonated beverage which is flavoured with oil of sassafras and oil of wintergreen.

Rope. Bacteria of the type B, measentericus and B, subtilis are found on wheat and thence in flour. These organisms form spores that can survive baking and then a represent in the bread. Under the right conditions of warmth and moisture the spores will germinate and the mass of bacteria convert the bread into sticky, yellowish patches which can be pulled out in to rope-like threads-hence the term ropy bread. The bacterial growth gets inhibited by acid substances. Can also occur in milk and carbonated beverages.

Rose-gottlieb Test. For fat in milk, accurate gravimetric method, by extracting the fat with solvent.

Rose Hips. Refers to the fruit of the rose; a rich source of vitamin C from which rose hip syrup is prepared.

Rose Hip Syrup. Extract of rose hip with added sugar. It is used as source of vitamin C-150mg per 100mg.

Rosemary. A bushy shrub, Rosmarinus officinalis. It is cultivated commercially for its essential oil, used in medicine and perfumery.The dried leaves are used to flavour soups, sauces and meat.

Rotary Lonvre Dryer. Hot air passes through a moving bed of the solid inside a rotating drum.

Roth-benedict Spirometer. Spirometer.

Ruox. Preparation of flour and butter for thickening gravies and sauces.

Royal Jelly. The term used for the food on which bee larvae are fed and which causes them to develop into queen bees. Richest known source of pantothenic acid (100µg per g dry weight): also contains vitamin B^6 and 2% of its dry weight is 10-hydroxy-delta-2-decenoic acid.

RPV. Abbreviation of relative protein value.

RO. Abbreviation of respiratory quotient.

Rubble Reel. Machine which is used for cleaning materials such as wheat. The material is fed into a long inclined reel made of perforated metal that rotates inside a frame. The perforations become large nearer the bottom, so that there occurs a graded sieving of the material as it passes down the reel.

Rubner Factors. Factors which are used to calculate the energy content of foods in kilocalories after allowing for losses of urinary nitrogen but not allowing for incomplete absorption, therefore greater than Atwater factors, protein 4.1, fat 9.3, carbohydrates 4.1.

Rum. A spirit which is distilled from fermented molasses. There are three main categories, Cuban, Jamaican and Dutch East Indies.

Rumen. Ruminating animals, like the cow, sheep and goat, have four stomachs, in distinction from monogastric animals, like man, pig, dog, and rat. These four are the rumen, or first stomach, where bacterial fermentation produces lower fatty acids, and whence the food is returned to the mouth for further mastication (chewing the cud), the reticulum, where further bacterial fermentation produces lower fatty acids, the omasum, and the abomasum or true stomach. The bacterial fermentation permits ruminants to get nourishment from grass and hay which cannot be digested by monogastric animals.

S

Saffron. Dried stigma of Crocus sativus (related to garden crocus). It is having glycoside picrocrocin, and colouring principles crocin and crocetin. Used as natural dyestuff (permitted food colour) and spice. Very soluble in water.

Sage. Refers to the dried leaf of the Dalmatian sage, Salvia officinalis, of the mint family, fragrant and spicy and is the most important herb used in the kitchen for flavouring meat and fish dishes and in poultry stuffing.

Sago. Starchy grains which are prepared from the pith of the sago plam (Metrozylon sago); almost pure starch free from protein.

Seithe. Polachius virens. Also termed as coley and coal fish. Apart from being eaten cooked, it is smoked, salted and dyed red, when it is similar to smoked salmon.

Sake. Japanese beer which is made from rice. Cooked whole rice grains are fèrmented with a yeast-like fungus culture for 10-14 days and stored in wooden barrels. Having about 17% alcohol, by volume. Also known as rice wine.

Salad Cream. Oil-in-water emulsion which is made from vegetable oil, vinegar, salt, spices, emulsified with egg yolk and thickened.

Salinometer. Or salimeter, or salometer. Hydrometer to measure concentration of salt solutions.

Salisbury Cure. Exclusive protein diet, supposed to cure or alleviate a number of disease.

Salisbury Steak. Similar to hamburger-minced lean beef mixed with bread, eggs, milk and seasonining, shaped into cakes and fried.

Saliva. Refers to secretion of the salivary glands in the mouth. There are three pairs of glands-parotid, submandibular and submaxillary. Dilute solution of the protein mucin and the enzyme amylase, with small quantities of urea, potassium thocyanate, sodium chloride and bicarbonate. One to 1.5 liter per day secreted of solution of 0.5% solids. The mucin lubricates the food, and the amylase hydrolyses starch to maltose.

Salivary Grands. Saliva.

Sally Lunn. Refers to a sweet, spongy, yeast cake which is named after a girl of that name who sold her tea cakes in the streets of Bath 1788.

Salmonella. Genus of bacteria of family Enterobacteriaceae. Common cause of food poisoning. It is found in egg from infected hens, sausages, etc. it can survive in brine and in the refrigerator. It gets destroyed by adequate heating.

Salt. Usually refers to sodium chloride, i.e. common salt or table salt (although any compound of acid and alkali is a salt).

Salt Content. Salt-free diets.

Salt-free Diets. More correctly these are diets low in (never completely free from) sodium but as most of the sodium of the diet is consumed as sodium chloride or salt, they are termed as low-salt diets. It is the sodium and not the chloride that is of importance.

Foods low in salt (0-2mg/100g) : sugar, flour, fruit, green vegetables, macaroni, nuts. Medium salt (50-100mg/100g) : chicken, fish, eggs, meat, milk. High salt (500-200mg/100g) : corned beef, bread, ham, bacon, kippers, sausages, cheese.

Saltlicks. An adequate intake of sodium chloride has been necessary to all animals. Grass is relatively poor in sodium, and its high potassium content induces excretion of sodium in the urine. This loss brings about a craving for sodium which is satisfied by natural or artificial saltlicks.

Saltpetre. (Bengal saltpetre). Potassium nitrate.

Sambol. Name a given to a curry of fairly solid consistency in India and other parts of the East.

Sami. Socially acceptable monitoring instrument. A small, heart rate counting apparatus which is used to estimate energy expenditure of human subjects.

Samp. Coarsely cut portions of maize with bran and germ partly removed.

Sapodilla. Refers to the fruit of the sapodilla tree (Achras sapota); size of a small apple, rough-grained, yellow to greyish pulp.

Chicle, the basis of chewing gum, made from the latex of the same tree.

Saponification. Refers to splitting of fat its constituent glycerol and fatty acids by boiling with alkali. The fatty acids will be present at the sodium salts, also called the sodium soaps.

Method of concentrating vitamin A from oils, because the vitamin does not saponify and can then get separated from the rest of the fat in the so-called non-saponifiable fraction. The latter also contains mineral oils and higher alcohols such as cholesterol.

Saponification Value. Use d with reference to fats as an indication of the nature (molecular weight) of the fatty acids present. It may be defined as the number of milligrams of potassium hydroxide required to saponify 1g of fat. Values greater than 200 are shortchain fatty acids; below 190 are of high molecular weight.

Saponins. Refer to group of substances that are found in plants and can produce a soapy lather with water. Extracted commercially from soapwort or soapbark and used as foam producer in beverage and fire extinguishers, as detergent and for emulsifying oils. Bitter in flavour.

There is a second group, the steroid saponins, which are cardiac active and find use as a starting material for the synthesis of sex hormones.

Saran. Generic name for thermoplastic materials which is made from polymers of vinylidine chloride. They are clear transparent films used for wrapping food, resistant to oils and chemicals; can be heat-shrunk on to the product.

Sarcosine. N-methyglycin. It is found in starfish and sea urchins; intermediate in the synthesis of antienzyme agents in toothpaste.

Sardine. Yound pilchard, Sardina (Clupea) pilchardus.

Sarsaparilla. Flavour which is prepared from oil of sassafras and oil of wintergreen or oil of sweet birch; used in a carbonated beverage.

Sassafras Oil. Used to flavour root beer and similar beverages, Main component has been safrole, believed to be a weak hepatic carcinogen and banned in some countries.

Sauerkraut. Obtained by lactic fermentation of shredded cabbage. In the presence of 2-3% salt, acid-forming bacteria thrive and convert sugars in the cabbage into acetic and lactic acids, which then act as preservatives.

Sausage. Chopped met, mostly beef or pork which are seasoned with salt and spices, mixed with cereal (usually wheat rusk prepared from crumbed unleavened biscuits) and packed into casings made from the connective tissue of animal intestines or cellulose.

There are six main types—fresh, smoked, cooked, smoked and cooked, semi-dry and dry. Frankfurters, Bologna, polish and Berliner sausages are made from cured meat and are smoked and cooked. Thuringer, soft salami, mortadella and soft cervelat are semi-dry sausages. Pepperoni, chorizos, dry salami-dry cervelat are slowly dried to a hard texture.

Sausage Casings. Natural casings are prepared from hog intestines for fresh frying sausages, and from sheep intestines for chipolatas and frankfurters. Skinless sausages are prepared in cellulose casing, which is then peeled off.

Saute. Toss in hot fat without browing (saute potatoes

usually cooked first and browned).

Saveloy. Highly seasoned smoked sausage; the addition of salt petre causes to the bright red colour. Originally a sausage made from pig; brains.

Savory. Plant with strongly flavoured leaves used as seasoning in sauces, soups, salad dishes. Summer savory is an animal, Satureja hortensis; winter savory is a perennial, Satureja montana. The plants are cut down at flowering time and dried for lalter use.

Scald. Defect occurring in stored apples, involving formation of brown patches on the skin, with browning and softening of the tissues underneath. Due to accumulation of gases given off during ripening.

Schardinger's Enzyme. The same as xanthine oxidase. It oxidises a whole range of aldehydes to acids, and also xanthine and hypoxanthine to uric acid.

Schilling Test. Test for vitamin B_{12} nutritional status by measuring the urinary excretion of a dose of levelled B_{12} given orally accompained by large parenteral dose of non-labelled B_{12}.

Scombroid Poisoning. Caused by bacterial spoilage of scombroid family of fish-including tunny, mackerel, sardines. Because of the formation of histamine in relatively large amounts from the amino acid histidine in the fish muscle, by the organism Proteus morganil. Results include headache, palpitation, flushing and diarrhoea; poisoning has arisen from canned tuna and from smoked mackerel.

Scone. Refers to a variety of tea cake which was originally made from oatmeal and sour milk, in Scone, Scotlant.

SCP. Single cell protein.

Scrapple. Meat dish which is prepared from pork carcass trimmings. Maize meal, flour, salt and spices—cooked to a thick consistency.

Scrod. Young cod.

Scuppernong. Name of the most widely cultivated of the muscadine grapes. It is used chiefly in wine rather than as a desert grape.

Scurvy. Vitamin C.

Scurvy Grass. A herb, Cochlearia officinalis. It is recommended as far back as late sixteenth century as a remedy for scurvy.

Scutellum. Area which is surrounding the embryo of the cereal grain; scutellum plus embryo is the germ. Rich in vitamins.

SDS. Sucrose distearate.

SE. Starch equivalent.

Seaweed. Algae of interest as food. Irish moss, laver bread and kelp are eaten to some extent in different communities and serve as a mineral supplement in animal feed.

Secretin. Hormone which is secreted by the intestinal mucosa. It travels via the blood stream to the pancreas and stimulates this organ to secrete it is a small, basic polypeptide, destroyed by pepsin and trypsin, and therefore ineffective when given by mouth.

Sedoheptulose. A 7-carbon sugar. Also called sedoheptose.

Seitz Filter. Asbestos disc with pores so fine that they will not allow passage of bacteria; thus solutions filtered through a Seitz filter emerge sterile.

Selenium. Dietary essential, because it is part of the enzyme glutathinone peroxidase, but toxic in excess. Can replace vitamin E in some but not all its functions.

Semolina. Refers to the inner, granular, starchy endosperm of hard or durum when (not yet ground into flour). It is used to make pasta and semolina milk pudding.

Sequestrants. Substances that combine with a metal iron or acid radical and render it inactive, e.g. citrates, tartrates, phosphates, and various calcium salts.

Serendiptiy Berry. Dioscoreophyllum cumminsii. West African fruit with an extremely sweet taste. Active principle called monellin.

Serine. Refers to a non-essential amino acid; amino hyroxypropionic acid.

Serosal. In reference to the intestine, it implies the outer side of the intestinal wall, as distinct from the inner or mucosal side.

Serum. Clear liquid which is left after the protein has been clotted; reference both to blood and milk. The serum from the milk, occasionally referred to as lacto-serum, is whey.

Serum, Blood. Blood plasma without the fibrinogen. When blood clots, the fibrinogen gets converted to ribrin, which gets deposited in strands that trap the red cells and form the clot. The clear liquid that is exuded is the serum.

Sesame. Sesamim indicum. Tropical and sub-tropical plant, also known as sim-sim in East Africa and benniseed in West Africa. Seeds are small and, in most varieties, white; used whole in sweetmeats, in stews and to decorate cakes and bread, and for extraction of the oil.

Seville Orange. Spanish term for the bitter orange.

Sfumatrice. Machine which is used for obtaining the oil from the peel of citrus fruit. Based on the principle that the natural turgor of the oil sacs forces out oil when the peel is folded.

Shaddock. Alternative name for pomelo, Citrus grandis, from which grapefruit gets descrended.

Sharples Centrifuge. Continuous high-speed centrifuge (15000-30000 rev/min) consisting of vertical cylinder. It is used to separate liquids of different densities or to clarify by sedimenting solids.

Shashlik. Similar to shishkebab, omitting steeping the meat in wine, According to some recipes the same as shishkebab.

Shearling. Sheep 15-18 months old.

Shellfish, Edible. Include prawns, shrimps, lobsters, crayfish and crabs. Zoologically they are of the order Decapoda, sub-order Macrura (prawns, shrimps, lobsters and crayfish) and sub-order Brachyura (crabs).

Shishkebab. Lamb (although beef sometimes used) cut into cubes steeped in onion, gallic and wine for a few hours, impaled on a skewer; pieces of meat alternating with tomatoes, mushrooms, or pieces of eggplant, dusted with flour and then broiled.

Shortening. Refers to soft fats that produce a crisp, flakey effect in baked products. Lard is having the correct properties to a greater extent than any other single fat. Unlike oils, shortenings are plastic and disperse as a film through the batter and prevent the formation of a hard, tough mass. Shortenings get compounded from mixtures of fats or prepared by hydrogenation and are still called lard compounds or lard substitutes.

Shrimp. The pink shrimp commonly sold at fishmongers is Pandalus montagui.

Sialic Acid. Refers to a group of compounds derived from neuraminic acid which are constituents of certain mucoproteins in the tissues, they include acetyl and glycolyl neuraminic acids. Also called lactaminic and gynaminic acids.

Sialogogue. Substance that stimulates the flow of saliva.

Siderophilin. Or transferrin, an iron carbonate-protein complex, the form in which iron gets transported in the blood plasma.

Siderosis. Refers to the accumulation of the iron-protein complex, haemosiderin, in liver, spleen and bone marrow in cases of excessive red cell destruction and on diets exceptionally rich in iron. It is common among Bantu, apparently owing to intakes of about 100mg of iron daily from iron cooking pots and kaffir beer.

Sild. Young herring, Clupea harengus.

Sillica Gel. Drying agent.

Silicones. Organic compounds of silicon; in the food field they find use a s antifoaming agents, as semi-permanent glazes on baking tins and other metal containers, on non-sticking wrapping paper.

Silver. Not of interest in foods apart from its use in covering 'nonpareils'—the silver beads used to decorate confectionery. Present in traces in all plant and animal tissues but is having no function nor is enough ever absorbed to cause toxicity.

Single Cell Protein. Collective term used for biomass of bacteria, algae and yeast, and also (incorrectly) moulds, of potential use as animal or human food.

Sippet. A small piece of bread, fried or toasted which is served as a garnish to a mince or hash.

Sippy Diet. For peptic ulcer patients; hourly feeds of small quantities, 150ml of milk, cream or other milk food.

Sitapophasis. Refusal to eat as expression of metal disorder.

Sitology. Science of food (from the Greek sitos, food).

Sitomania. Maina for eating.

Sitophobia. Fear of food, also phagophobia.

Sitosterol. The main sterol which is found in vegetable oils. It is similar in structure to cholesterol with an extra ethyl group.

Sliwowitz. Plum brandy, originating in Yugoslavia. Some of the stones are included with the fruit and produce a characteristic bitter flavour from the hydrocyanic acid (0.008% HCN is present in the finished brandy).

Sole. Wild sour plum of the blackthorn (Prunus spinosa); almost only use is for the manufactured of sole gin.

SLR Factor. Streptococcus lactis factor.

Smoke Point. A term which is used with reference to frying oils; the temperature at which the decomposition products become visible (bluish smoke). The temperature varies with different fats and ranges between 160 and 260°C.

Smoking. Meat and fish are generally smoked after pickling to assist preservation and improve the flavour. Hard woods, oak, elm, and ash, produce a smoke having aldehydes, phenols and acids with a preservative action; surface dehydration also helps preservation.

Smorrebrod. Danish open sandwiches; literally means smeared bread.

SMS. Sucrose monostearate.

Smut. Refers to a group of fungi that attack wheat; includes loose or common smut (Ustilago tritici) and stinking smut or bunt (Tilletia tritict).

SN. Stereochemical numbering. It is used in nomenclature of lipids to indicate that the system of numbering the glycerol carbon atoms is being used in place of the DL system.

Snibbing. Topping and tailing of gooseberries.

Soapstock. In the refining of crude edible oils the free fatty acids are removed by agitation with alkali. The fatty acids settle to the bottom as alkali soaps and are termed as soapstock or 'foots'.

Soda Bread. Made from flour and whey, or butter milk, using sodium bicarbonate and acid in place of yeast. Common in Ireland.

Sodium. Refers to a dietary essential which is almost invariably satisfied by the normal diet. The body is having about 100g of sodium and the average diet contains 3-6g, equivalent to 10g of sodium chloride. The intake varies enormously in different individuals and the excretion varies accordingly.

Vegetables are relatively poor in sodium and rich in potassium. Animal foods are rich in sodium.

Sodium Chloride. Common salt-the commonest form in which sodium is consumed.

Sodium Glutamate. Glutamate, sodium.

Soft Drinks. Term used for non-alcoholic, usually fruit and fruit flavoured drinks. Various concentrations and preparations are termed squash, crush and cordial, which usually require dilution before drinking; others are ready-to-drink.

In the USA cider refers to unfermented apple-juice (a soft drink), while the fermented product is called hard cider.

Sol. A colloidal solution, i.e. a suspension of particles intermediate in size between molecule (as in a solution) and coarse particles (as in a suspension). A jelly-like sol is a gel.

Solanaceae. Family of plants including potato (solanum tuberosum), aubergine (S. melongena). Cape gooseberry (Physalisperuviana), tomato (Lycopersicon esculentum).

Solanine. Refers to heat-stable toxic glycoside of the alkaloid solanidine, found in small amounts of potatoes, and large and sometimes toxic amounts in sprouts and in skin when potatoes become green through exposure to light. 20mg solanine per 100g fresh weight of potato tissue is accepted as the upper limit. Causes gastrointestinal disturbances and certain neurological disorders; in vitro it inhibits cholinesterase.

Solids not-fat. Refers to the solids of milk excluding the fat, i.e., protein, lactose and salts. SNF acts as an index of milk quality and is determined by measuring the specific gravity in the lactometer.

Normal specific gravity is 1.0032 at 60°F (15.5°C).

Percentage total solids = 0.25 × SG+1.2 × percentage fat 0.14.

Sorbet. Sherbet.

Sorbic Acid. Formula $CH_2CH{=}CH{=}CHCH{=}CHCOOH$. It is used to inhibit selectively growth of yeasts and moulds (not bacteria). Metabolised in the same way as the naturally occurring caproci acid (of butter) and so generally held to be harmless.

It finds use in margarine (0.05%), fruit juice (0.02%) sauces, cheese, jam, flour confectionery (0.1%).

Potassium sorbate is more soluble in water. Occurs in certain berries as the free acid and the delta-lactone; first claimed as antimycotic in 1945.

Is active as the undissociated acid and therefore the concentration for preservation is related to the acidity of food. Effective at pH 5.0-7.0.

Sorbitol. Six-carbon sugar alcohol which is formed by the reduction of fructose; old names glycitol and glucitol. Although it is metabolised in the body with the liberation of 4 kcal per gram, it gets absorbed from the intestine only slowly and is tolerated by diabetics. It occurs in plum, apricot, cherry and apple; used in place of sucrose to make jam suitable for diabetics; 60% as sweet as sucrose.

Sorenson Titration. A method of titrating amino acids and ammonium salts by adding formaldehyde, which reacts with the amino groups, and titrating the carboxyl groups (or acidic radical of the ammonium salt).

Sorghum. Sorghum vulgare. Refers to a cereal that thrives in semi-arid regions; important human food in tropical Africa, Central and N. India and China. Sorghum produced in the USA and Australia is used for animal feed. Also known as kaffir corn (in South Africa), guinea corn (in West Africa), jowar (in India) and millo maize. The white grain variety in eaten as meal, red grained has a bitter taste and is used for beer; sugar syrup is obtained from the crushed stems of the sweet sorghum.

Sorghum syrup. Refers to the concentrated juice from a sweet variety of sorghum.

Souse. To steep or cook a food like herring in vinegar or white wine.

Soxhiet. An apparatus which is used for the extraction of solids. It is mostly used for the extraction of fat. The solid is contained in a 'thimble' and is percolated by fresh solvent continuously. The fat-laden solvent siphons over into a flask from which is gets boiled off the be repercolated, while the fat gets left in the flask.

Soya. Refers to a bean (Glycine max) of importance as a source of both oil and protein. The protein is of high biological value, higher than that of many other vegetable proteins, and is of great value for animal and human food.

When raw it is having trypisin inhibitor destroyed by heat.

Soybean Curd. Precipitate from soybean milk.

Soybean Flour. Dehulled, ground soya bean. The unheated material, has been a rich source of amylase and proteinase and is useful as a baking aid. The heated material has no enzymic activity but is a valuable food. There is about 25% carbohydrate in the bean, of which 12% is polysaccharide (dextrins, galactans and pentosans) and 12.5% sugars (6% sucrose, 5% stachyose and 1.5% raffinose).

Soybean milk. Extract of the bean.

Soy Sauce. The fermented soya bean commonly eaten in China and Japan. Traditionally the bean, often mixed with wheat, is fermented with Aspergillus oryzae over a period of 1-3 years. The modern process is carried out a high temperature or in an autoclave for a short time.

Specific Dynamic Action. The term which is applied to the increase in metabolism (as indicated by heat output) following ingestion of food. In modern terminology it is referred to as thermogenesis or the thermic effect, though to be due to stimulation of brown fat. Possible means whereby constant body weight is maintained despite variations in food intake.

Spectrophotometer. An optical instrument that measures the amount of light absorbed at any particular wavelength. It is used extensively to measure substances that have specific absorption in the infrared or ultraviolet range, or are coloured, or can react to form colour derivatives. Similar in this way to the absorptiometer.

Spelt. Coarse type of wheat which is mainly used as cattle feed.

Spent Wash. Liquor remaining in the whisky still after distilling the spirit. A source of unidentified growth factors detected by chick growth. When dried is known as distillers dried solubles.

Sphinogomyelins. Complex phosphatides which are found in brain and nerve tissue and as part of cell structure; composed of the base sphingosine plus fatty acids, phosphoric acid and choline.

Spices. Distinguished from herbs only in that part instead of the whole of the aromatic plant is meant, such as root, stem, seeds.

Originally these are used to mask putrefactive flavours. Some have preservative effect because of their essential oils, e.g. cloves, cinnamon and mustard.

Consumed in too small a quantity to provide any nutrients, except possibly for curry powder, which contains 22mg iron per ounce.

Spinach. Leaves of Spinacia oleracea. It is a rich source of carotene and vitamin C; also contains oxalic acid, which makes calcium insoluble and non-available.

Spirits. Prepared by distillation of yeast fermentation liquors, subsequently diluted. Alcohol content, w/v, of brandy, gin, rum, whisky, 31.7% (termed 70 degrees proof), with traces of nitrogen, minerals and sugars.

Spirit, Silent. Highly purified alcohol, or neutral spirit. It is distilled from any fermentable material.

Spirometer. (respirometer). An apparatus which is used to measure the amount of oxygen consumed (and in some instances the amount of carbon dioxide produced) from which to calculate the energy expended (indirect calorimetry). There are several types, including the Benedict-Roth spirometer, the Kofranyl-Michaelis spirometer and the integrating motor pneumotacho graph (IMP).

Spirulina. Blue-green alga which can make use of atmospheric nitrogen; eaten for centuries round Lake Chad in N. Africa and in Mexico.

Spores. In relation to bacteria, they are the resting state; thick walled, highly resistant to damage by heat. Under suitable conditions they germinate to produce bacteria.

Spart. Sprattus (Clupea sprattus), related to the herring; found in brisling.

Spray Dryer. An equipment in which material to be dried is sprayed as a fine mist into a hot-air chamber and falls to the bottom as dry powder. Period of heating is very brief and so damage is avoided. Dried powder consists of hollow particles of low density. Widely applied to many foods (e.g., milk and pharmaceuticals).

Sprue. Refers to the disease in which the villi of the small intestine are atrophied and food is incompletely absorbed, followed consequently by undernutrition and weight loss, in tropical sprue.

Sprue, Tropical. Name given (by Dutch in Java) to tropical disease of unknown origin which is characterised by fatty diarrhoea and sore mouth, with signs of undernutrition due to poor absorption of nutrients.

Squaliene. A hydrocarbon, $C_{30}H_{50}$ which is found in liver of shark and rat. It is a possible intermediate in the synthesis of cholesterol in the body.

Stabilisers. Also emulsifying agents. Substances that are able to stabilise emulsions of fat and water, e.g., gums, agar, egg albumin, cellulose ethers; used to produce the texture of meringues and marshmallow, lecithin for crumb-softening in bread and confectionery, glyceryl monostearate and polyoxyethylene stearate for crumb-softening.

Stachyase. Enzyme that is able to hydrolyse the tetrasaccharide stachyose to fructose and mannosaccharide consisting of glucose and two molecules of galactose. Occur in the digestive juices of crustaceans and molluscs.

Stachyose. Tetrose sugar which is composed of two units of galactose and one each of fructose and glucose. It is not hydrolysed in the human digestive tract and passes to the large intestine, where it gets fermented by bacteria. Present in soya beans, some other legumes, including lupins, and the tuber of Stachys tubifera; gives rise to the flatulence commonly associated with eating beans. Also known as mannotetrose and lupeose.

Stackburn. Name assigned to the deterioration in colour and quality of canned foods which have not been sufficiently cooled after canning and then stored in stacks which slowly.

Staling. As applied to baked products as such bread, is thought to be due to the slow passage of water from the starch to other components of the bread. It is assumed that anti-staling agents function by forming an insoluble coating round the starch granules, which slow down the passage of water.

Staple Food. The principal food, e.g., wheat, rice, maize, etc.

Starch. Complex polysaccharide which is composed unit of glucose. It consists of about one-quarter amylose and three quarters amylo-pectin; the form which carbohydrate is stored in the plant, and does not occur in animal tissue. (Glycogen is sometimes termed as animal starch).

All starches are broken down by acid hydrolysis, or during digestion, first to maltose and then glucose, but the various starches like potato, maize, cereal, arrow root, sago, etc., have different structures.

Starch Equivalent. Refers to a measure of the energy value of animal feedingstuffs; the number of parts of pure starch that would be equivalent to 100 parts of the ration as a source of energy. It is determined by direct feeding experiments or may be calculated from the formula : SE per 100lb = 0.44 × digestible protein plus 2.41 × digestible fat plus digestible carbohydrate plus fibre.

Protein is having SE 0.94, crude fibre 1.0 ether extract of oilseeds 2.4 llb starch equivalent has net energy value of 1071 kcal : 1 kg = 9.9 MJ.

Starches, Waxy. Those a high percentage of amylopectin : they do not form rigid gels when gelatinished but soft pastes.

Starch, Modified. Starch which altered by physical or chemical treatment to give special properties of value in food processing, e.g., change in gel strength, flow properties, colour, clarity, stability of the paste.

Acid-modified starch-acid treatment decreases the viscosity of the paste (used in sugar confectionery, e.g., gum drops, jelly beans.)

Oxidised starch-peroxide, permanganate, chlorine, etc., change viscosity, clarity and stability of the paste (major use is outside the food industry).

Derivatised starch-chemical derivatives like others and esters show properties such as reduced gelatinisation in hot water and greater stability to acids and alkalies ('inhibited' starch); useful where food has to withstand he at treatment, as in canning or in acid foods. Further degrees of treatment can result in starch being unaffected by boiling water losing its gel-forming properties.

Starch, Pregelatinised. Raw starch does not form a paste with cold water and therefore needs cooking if it is to be used as a food thickening agent. Pregelatinised starch, mostly maize starch, has been cooked and dried. It finds use in instant puddings, pie-filings, soup mixes, salad dressings, sugar confectionery, as binder in meat products. Nutritional value the same as that of the original starch.

Starter. Culture of bacteria which are used to inoculate or start growth in, e.g. milk for cheese production, or butter to develop the flavour, or any fermentation.

Steam Baking. In baking an even temperature is maintained in the oven by using closed pipes through which steam circulates. This is sometimes erroneously believed to mean that the bread is baked in live steam.

Steaic Acid. Refers to the saturated long-chain fatty acid with 18 carbon atoms-octadecenoic acid, $C_{17}H_{35}COOH$. It is present in most animal and vegetable fats in the triglycerides. Used in pharmacy and cosmetics.

Steatorrhoea. Excess of fat in the stools. May occur due to lack of bile, lack of lopase in the digestive juice, or defective absorption of fat. Treatment by feeding low-fat diet.

Steer. Bull castrated when very young; if castrated after reaching maturity, known as a stag.

Stercobilin. Refers to one of the brown pigments of the faeces; formed from the bile pigments, which, in turn, gets formed as breakdown products of the haemolgobin of obsolete red blood cells.

Stereoisomerism. Occurs when compounds are having the same molecular formula, and the same structural formula, but with the atoms arranged differently in space. There are two subdivisions, namely, optical isomerism and geometrical isomerism.

Sterile. Free from all micro- organisms-bacteria, moulds and yeasts. When foods are sterilised, as in canning, they are preserved indefinitely, as they are protected from recontamination in the can, and also from chemical and enzymic deterioration.

Sterilisation, Cold. Applied to preservation with sulphur dioxide or with ionising radiation.

Sterility, Commercial. Term applied to canned foods which are not sterile but which will not spoil during storage, due to the high acid content of the food, or the presence of pickling salts, or a high concentration of sugar.

Sterols. Alcohols which are derived from the steroids. Include cholesterol, widely distributed in animal tissue, including brain and egg yolk; coprosteral in faeces; ergosterol in yeast, which is the precursor for the synthetic vitamin D_2 : and sitosterol and stigmasterol in plants.

Stevioside. Refers to the naturally occurring glucoside of steviol, a steroid derivative, which is 300 times as sweet as source. Isolated from leaves of Paraguayan shrub, Stevia rebaudianayerpa dulce.

Stew. To cook foods in an enclosed pan; temperature below boiling point, about 90°C (195°F). Such slow cooking has been useful for low-quality meat (rich in connective tissue), because it slowly breaks down the connective tissue to gelatian and so softens the meat.

Stickwater. Refers to the aqueous fraction from pressing cooked fish in the manufacture of fish meal. Contains amino acids, vitamins and minerals, and is added to animal feed or mixed back with the fish meal and dried. Also known as fish solubles.

Stilboestrol. Synthetic substance having potent activity as female sex hormone : widely used clinically and for food production (for chemical caponisation of cockerels and to stimulate the growth of cattle).

Stiparogenic. Foods that tend to bring about constipation.

Stiparolytic. Foods that tend to prevent or relieve constipation.

Stobb. Strawberry stalk.

Stockfish. Unsalted fish that has been dried naturally in air and sunshine, Contains 12-15% water, and 1 lb is made from 4-1/2 lb of fresh fish.

Stock; Meat Vegetable, Bone Stock. Refers to liquid in

which the meat or bone or vegetable, or a mixture of these, has been boiled until most of the water-soluble matter has been extracted.

Meat and bone are having collagen, which is converted into gelatin by prolonged boiling; hence, the stock may set to a gel on cooling. The main nutritive value of stock is the mineral content.

Stork process. The name given to the process of ultra-high temperature sterilisation of milk which is followed by sterilsation again in side the bottle.

Stout. So-called milk sout merely has added lactose (milk sugar).

Stradin. A substance isolated from bain tissue which dries in long stands. It is composed of fatty acid, sphingosine, carbohydrate and a small proportion of neuraminic acid.

Strawberry. Fruit of Fragaria species, a perennial herb of American origin, introduced into Europe about 1600, 40-90mg vitamin C per 100g : trace of carotene.

Alpine strawberry is Fragaria vesca semperflorens, a variety of the European wild strawberry.

Strepogenin. Name given to a peptide-like fraction from natural source. It is claimed to be essential for micro-organisms and higher animals. The need for special peptides for the latter has not been confirmed.

Streptococcal. Food poisoning.

Streptococcus Lactis Factor. Refers to a fermentation product of the mould Rhizopus nigricans, known as rhizopterin, which is essential to S. lactics R. Related to folic acid.

Streptokinase. Proteoyltic enzymes which is prepared from haemolytic streptococci. Used clinically to liquefy thick pus empyemata and to remove the fibrin clot covering wounds. Streptodornase is a similar enzyme preparation that attacks pus cells.

Struvite. Refers to small crystals ormagnesium ammonium phosphate which occasionally form in canned fish-resemble broken glass.

Substrate. In relation to enzymes, refers to the substance on which the enzyme acts. Thus, the substrate for the enzyme amylase is starch, which is hydrolysed to maltose. Substrate can also mean the medium on which micro-organisms grow.

Subtilin. Antibiotic which is isolated from a strain of Bacillus subtilis grown on a medium containing asparagine. It finds use as a food preservative as it reduces the thermal resistance of spores and is effective against thermophilic flat sours; thus, subtilin permits a reduction in the processing time.

Succotash. Stew of green maize and Lima beans (butter beans), an American-Indian dish.

Success Entericus. Intestinal juice.

Suchar. Activated carbon which is used to decolorise solutions.

Sucrose. Cane sugar or beet sugar. A disaccharide which is composed of a molecule of glucose linked to one of fructose; these two monosaccharides are formed by the hydrolysis of sucrose. Refined white sugar is close to 100% pure and is having no minerals or vitamins.

Sucrose Esters. Di-and trilaurates and mono-and distearates of sucrose. These are used as emulsifiers, wetting agents and surface active agents e.g. for washing fruits and vegetables, as anti-spartering agents, anti-foam agents and anti-staling or crumb-softening agents.

Suet. Fat which is prepared from the kidneys of oxen and sheep.

Sugar. Although the term has been commonly used to refer to table sugar or sucrose, there have been a large number of sugars, e.g. fruit sugar (fructose), grape (glucose), which are monosaccharides; malt sugar (maltose), milk sugar (lactose), which are disaccharides; and also higher multiples.

Table sugar (sucrose) is extracted from the sugar beet or sugar cane, concentrated and refined.

Sugar Beet. Beta Vulgaris subsp, cicla. It is the most important source of sugar (sucrose) in temperature countries; contains 15-20% sugar, biennial related to the garden beetroot but with white, conical roots.

Sugar Cane. The plant, Saccharum officinarum, from the juice of which sugar is prepared.

Sugar Doctor. So as to prevent the crystallisation or 'graining' of sugar in sugar confectionary, a substance called the sugar doctor or candy doctor is added. This may be a weak acid, such as cream of tartar which 'invert' part of the cane sugar during the boiling, or invert sugar or starch syrup.

Sugaring, of Dried Fruits. Refers to a type of deterioration of dried fruit on storage, most frequently on prunes and figs. A sugary substance appears on the surface or under the skin, consisting of glucose and fructose, with traces of citric and malic acids, lysine, asparagine and aspartic acid. When occurring under the skin of prunes, it is termed as 'red sugar'.

Sugar Maple. Acer saccharum; the sap gets evaporated down to a syrup, maple syrup and crystallised to sucrose, maple sugar.

Sugar Palm. Arenga saccharifera; grows wild in Malaysia and Indonesia. Sugar (sucrose) is obtained from the sap.

Sugar Tolerance. Glucose tolerance.

Sulpha Drugs. Group of synthetic drugs which are derived from sulphanilamide (or aminobenzenesulphonamide) used to combat bacterial infection. Sulfanilamide itself functions as an anti vitamin to baceteria, as it inhibits the uptake of para-amino benzoic acid, an essential nutrient. The drugs include sulphapyridine, sulphadiazine, sulphathiazole, etc.

Sulphate. The mineral sulphur is found in foods and in the body in two main forms, (1) as sulphate-salts of sulphuric acid, and (2) in the amino acids methionine and cystine.

Sulphur. An element that is part of the amino acids cystine and methionine and is therefore present in all proteins. It is also part of the molecules of vitamin B_1 and biotin. Apart from its presence as part of these compounds, there appears to be no dietary need for sulphur in any other form and no deficiency has ever been observed, although it has been essential for plants.

Sulphur Amino Acids. Cysteine and methionine; methionine is essential but can be partially replaced by cysteine, so the amounts of the two in a protein food are usually added together.

Sulphur Dioxide. Used in solution (sulphurous acid) as a preservative for sausage meat, liquid glucose, fruit, fruit pulp and juices, etc. One major advantage is that it gets driven off by boiling. Stabilises vitamin C but damages vitamin B_1.

Sulphuring. Preservation by sulphur dioxide.

Sulphur in Urine. Three groups of sulphur compounds get excreted : inoraganic sulphates (sodium, potassium, calcium, magnesium, and ammonium), organic sulphates (sulphuric esters of phenolic compounds), neutral (thiosulphates, thiocyanates, mercapturic acids, urochrome).

Sultanas. Made by drying the golden sultana grapes (Turkey, Greece, Australia, and South Africa); the bunches are dipped in alkali, washed, sulphured and dried. Sultanas of the European type produced in the USA are called seedless raisins.

Sunflower. Helianthus annuus. Seed which is used as source of edible oil, rich in polyunsaturated fatty acids; residual oilcake used for animal feed. Seeds also eaten raw.

Sunlight Flavour. Name given to unpleasant flavours developing in foods after exposure to sunlight. In milk it is said to be due to the breakdown of methionine in the presence of vitamin B_2 in beer due to a change in the bitter principles from the hops.

Superglycerinated Fats. Normal fats are triglycerides, i.e. three molecules of fatty acid to each molecule of glycerol. Mono- and diglycerides are known as superglycerinated.

Glyceryl monostearate (GMS) is solid at room temperature, flexible and non-greasy; used as a protective coating for foods, as plasticiser for softening the crumb of bread, to reduce spattering in frying fats, as emulsiter and stabiliser.

Glyceryl mono-oleate (GMS) is semi-liquid at room temperature.

Surface Area. Refers to heat loss from the body, and therefore basal metabolism, is related to surface area. Calculated by formula of Du Bosis or Meeh.

Du Bois : Area (cm^2) = weight (kg) to power of 0.425 × height ((cm) to power of 0.725) × 71.84.

Meeh : Area = 11.9 × weight to power of 2/3.

Surfactants. Refers to the surface active agents which are hydrophilic or have hydrophilic and hydrophobic portions of their structure and so have affinity for both fats and water and act as emulsifiers. There find use in baked goods, as wetting agents for powders, to clean and peel fruits and vegetables, and in comminuted meat products.

Sweat. Solution of salt (about 0.3%), urea 0.03% lactate 0.07%. It varies in composition but hypotonic to blood plasma.

Swede. Root of Brassica rutabaga or Swedish turnip : called rutabaga in the USA.

Sweeteners, Bulk. Used to replace sucrose and glucose syrups. One example is hydrogenated glucose syrup, in which the free aldehyde groups of glucose units are reduced to sorbitol by catalytic hydrogenation; effectively a mixture of glucose and sorbitol. It finds use in soft drinks and sugar confectionery, and in some diabetic foods as a partial substitute for sorbitol; 70-80% as sweet as sucrose.

Sweeteners. Non-nutritive. The sweetening agents which are not sugars and have no food value, as saccharin and cyclamate.

Sweetening Agents. There are three groups:

(1) The sugars, of which the commonest is sucrose. Fructose has 173% of the sweetness of sucrose; glucose, 74%; maltose, 33%; and lactose, 16%.

(2) Synthetic non-nutritive sweeteners such as

saccharine (550 times as sweet as sucrose), dulcin (250 times), sucaryl (30 times), p4000 (4000 times)-under individual headings.

(3) Various other chemicals such as glycerol and glycine (70% as sweet as sucrose), and certain peptides.

Swells. Applied to infected canned foods when gases produced by fermentation inside the can cause the ends to swell.

Syllabub. Also sillabub, Elizabethan dish made of milk or cream mixed with wine or brandy, sweetened and whipped.

Syneresis. Oozing of liquid from gel when cut and allowed to stand (e.g. jelley or baked custard).

Synthalin. Decamethylene-diguanidine. It lowers blood sugar and used experimentally in the treatment of diabetes, but is toxic.

Syrup. Refers to a solution of sugar which may be from a variety of sources such as maple, corn sorghum, and stages in refining such as top syrup, refiners and sugar syrup.

T

Tafia. Spirit which is similar to rum made from sugar cane.

Takadiastase. Or koji, an enzyme preparation which is produced by growing the fungus Aspergillus oryzae on bran, leaching the culture mass with water and precipitating with alcohol.
Having a mixture of enzymes, largely diastatic : used for the preparation of starch hydrolysates.

Tallow, Rendered. Beef or mutton fat prepared from parts other than the kidney, by heating with water in an autoclave. When pressed, separates to a liquid fraction, oleo oil, used in margarine, and a solid fraction, oleostearin, used for soap and candles.

Tamales. Flat, Mexican, cornmeal pancakes which are similar to tortillas, rolled around spiced met or fish or fruit.

Tamarind. Leguminous tree. Tamarindus indica; with pods containing seeds embedded in brown pulp, eaten fresh and used in seasonings and curries.

Tammy. Cookery term meaning to strain through a lime woollen cloth-a tammy cloth.

Tangelo. Ground, dried residue from slaughter house excluding all the useful tissues.

Tannia (also tanier). Corn of Xanthosoma sagittifulium; known as new cocoyam in West Africa and as yautia; same family as taro.

Tanins. Any polyphenolic substances with molecular weight greater than 500. It is classified as hydrolysable (to yield sugar it value and phenolcarboxylci acid) and condensed of compound tannis, which are polymeric flavonoids (also called catechin tannis).

These occur in dark-coloured sorghum, carbob bean, unripe fruits, tea; give an astringent effect in the mouth; precipitate proteins and used to clarify beer and wines. Also called tannic acid and gallotannin.

Tansy. Tanacetum vulgare. Leaves and young shoots which are used from flavouring puddings and omelettes. Tansy cakes made with eggs and young leaves used to be eaten at Easter. Tansy tea made by infusing the herb formerly used as tonic and for intestinal worms. Root, preserved in honey or sugar, was used for gout.

Tapioca. A starch which is prepared from the root of the cassava plant. The starch paste is heated to burst the granules, then dried either in globules resembling sago or in flakes. The term is also used of starch in general, as in manioc tapioca and potato flour tapioca.

Topioca-macaroni. Refers to a mixture of 80-90 parts tapioca flour, with 10-12 parts of peanut flour, or tapioca, peanut, semolina, 60 : 15 : 25, baked into shapes resembling rice grains or macaroni shapes; developed in India. Also termed as synthetic rice.

Taro. Corn of colocasia esculenta and C. antiquorum. It is called eddo or dasheen in West Indies, old cocoyam in West Africa.

Tarragon. Refers to the tried leaves and flowering tops of the bushy perennial plant Artemisia dracunculus. Having an anise-like flavour and has been used to flavour vinegar, and pickles, and is one of the ingredients of fines herbes.

Tarragon vinegar is made by steeping the fresh herb in white wine vinegar and is used in making sauce tartare and French mustard.

Tarter Emetic. Potassium antimony tartrate. It produces inflammation of the gastrointestinal mucosa and used to be used as an emetic.

Tartaric Acid. A dibasic acid, dihydroxysuccinin COOHCHOHCHOHCOOH. It is found in fruits, the chief source are grapes; used in preparing lemonade, added to jams when the fruit is not sufficiently acidic (citric acid also used) and in baking powder.

Tartar emetic is the potassium antimonyl salt, and Rochelle salt is potassium sodium tartrate.

Tartrazine. Yellow colour allowed in food in most countries; trisodium slat of 5-hydroxy-1-p-sulphophehyl azopyrazole-3-carboxylic acid.

Tartronat. Salt of tartronic (or hydroxymalonic) acid. Suggested as coenzyme in the decarboxylation of oxalosuccinic acid in the citric acid cycle and also claimed as a dietary essential for the rate but not confirmed.

Taste. Organoleptic.

Taste Buds. Situated having on the tongue; about 9000 elongated cells ending minute hairlike processes, the gustatory hairs.

Tea. Prepared from the young leaves, leaf buds and internodes of varieties of Camellia sinensis.

Green tea is dried without involving further treatment. Black tea is fermented (actually an oxidation) before drying; Oolong tea is slightly fermented.

Among the black teas, Flowering Pekoe is made from the top leaf buds, Orange Pekoe from first opened leaf, Pekoe from third leaves, and Sourchong from next leaves.

Teaseed Oil. Oil from the seed of Thea sasangua which is cultivated in China. It is used as salad oil and for frying; similar in properties to olive oil.

Teff. Millet-like cereal grain; major protein of the diet of Ethiopia.

Teg. Two-year-old sheep.

Tempen. Soya bean which is fermented by a fungus eaten in Indonesia.

Tenderiser. Usually refers to the enzyme papin, when used to tenderise meat. Weak acids like vinegar and lemon juice and 2% sodium chloride also tenderise meat.

Tenderometer. Instrument which is used to measure the

stage of maturity of peas to determine whether they are ready for canning. Measures the force required to effect a shearing action.

Tepary Bean. Phaseolus acutifolius, also known as Mexican haricot bean, frijole and pinto. It is able to grow during drought.

Tequila. Distilled liquor which is obtained from a fermented mash made from the cultivated cactus, Agave tequilana; 90-100 degrees proof; common in Mexico.

Mescal has been similar but made from the mescal agave, which grows wild and is much cheaper.

Teratogen. A substance which is able to deform the fetus in the womb and so induce birth defects.

Terpenses. Refer to the components of the essential oils of citrus fruits; hydrocarbons of the general formula $C_{10}H_{16}$; also sesquiterpenes, $C_{15}H_{24}$. Include limonene, alpha, beta, and gamma terpinene, alpha and beta phellandrene. Limonene is 90% of oil of orange.

Although terpenses constitute 90-95% of citrus oils, they are not responsible for the characteristic flavour, and as they readily oxidise and polymerise to produce unpleasant flavours, they are removed from citrus oils by distillation or solvent extraction, leaving the so-called terpeneless oils.

Terramycin. Antibiotic which is isolated in 1950 from streptomyces rimosus. Now known as oxytetracyline.

Testa. In reference to cereal grains, the testa refers to a fibrous layer between the pericarp and the inner aleurone layer.

Tetany. Oversenstivity or motor nerves to stimuli; particularly affects face, hands and feet. Caused by reduction in the level of ionised calcium in the blood stream and can accompany serve rickets.

Tetracyclines. Refers to the group of closely related antibiotics, tetracycline, oxytetracyline (aureomycin). The last two finds use in some countries for preserving food and, when added to animal feed at the rate of a few mg per ton, improve growth.

Of special use for eviscerated poultry; the bird is dipped in solution of 10 ppm, and, when stored at 34-37°F, shelf life gets extended from 10-14 to 17-21 days. 2ppm left in the poultry, much reduced on cooking.

Also of great value in extending the storage life of fresh fish by 2-3 days, by adding 5 ppm antibiotic to the ice or chilled water, or by dipping fillets into water containing 2-20ppm.

Tetraenoic Acid. Fatty acid having four double bonds, e.g. arachidonic acid.

Tetraodontin Poisoning. Get caused by fish to Tetraodontidal family (puffer fish) and amphibia of Salamandridae family, due to toxins in the entrails (Japan).

Tewfikose. Name given to a sugar which was isolated from a sample of buffalo milk obtained from Egypt in 1892. Later it was found to be an artefact; named after Tewfik Bey Pasha, Governor of Egypt.

Texture. Refers to the combination of physical properties perceived by senses of kinaesthesis (musicle-nerve endings), touch (including mouth feel), sight and hearing.

Textured Vegetable Protein. Refers to spun or extruded vegetable protein made to simulate meat.

Texture Profile. Organoleptic analysis of the complex of food in terms of mechanical, geometrical, fat and moisture content characteristics, including the order in which they appear from the first bite to complete mastication.

Theine. Alternative name for caffeine.

Theobromine. Dimethylxanthine. An alkaloid which occurs in cocoa in amounts ranging between 0.8 and 1.3% (together with caffeince trimethylxanthine, 0.140-0.7%).

Therapetic Diets. Those formulated to treat disease or metabolic disorder.

Thermisation. Heat treatment, less severe than pasteurisation e.g., heat treatment of milk for cheese-making whereby the number of organisms is diminished.

Thermoduric. Bacteria that are heat resistant but not

thermophilic. They are found in milk. They survive pasteurisation temperatures but do not develop at them. Usually not pathogens but indicative of insanitary conditions.

Thermopeeling. Refers to a method of peeling tough-skinned fruits in which the fruit is rapidly passed through an electric furnance at about 900°C then sprayed with water.

Thermophiles. Bacteria that prefer temperatures of 55°C (131°F) and above; can tolerate temperatures up to 75-80°C (167-176°F). Some strains reported to survive boiling 24 hours at ph 6.1.

Thermophilic bacteria are responsible for spontaneous combustion in hay stacks.

Thiamin. Vitamin B_1.

Thiaminase. An enzyme which is present in many species of fish. It hydrolyses thiamin and can therefore cause vitamin B_1 deficiency.

Thiochrome. Compound to which vitamin B_1 can get oxidised (for example, by potassium ferricyanide) and which gives a strong blue fluorescence in ultraviolet light. This used as an assay of the vitamin.

Threonine. Refers to a essential amino acid; the latest of the amino acids to get discovered, 1935; amino hydroxybutyric acid.

Thrombin. Plasma protein involved in coagulation of the blood, which see.

Thrombokinase. Or thromboplastin. It gets liberated from damaged tissue and blood plalteles; converts prothrombin to thrombin in coagulation of the blood which see.

Thunberg Tube. A test-tube which is carrying a curved hollow stopper. It is used to hold one of the reactants; the whole tube can be evacuated through a side-arm. It is used to study oxidation reactions where it becomes necessary to keep the reactants separate until the oxygen has been removed from the system.

Thuricide. Name used for a living culture of Bacillus

thuringensis which is harmless to mean but kills off insect pests. Known as a microbial insecticide. Used to treat certain foods and fodder crops to destroy pests like corn earworm, flour moth, tomato fruit worm, cabbage looper, etc. The bacillus is mass produced and stored like a chemical.

Thyroxine. Hydroxyphenyl-tetra-iodotyrosine. An hormone from the thyroid gland which gets converted into the more active tri-iodothyroine in the tissues.

Tin. A dietary essential for rats but is so widely distributed in foods that no deficiency has been reported in man. In the absence of oxygen tin is resistant to corrosion; hence, widely used in tinned cans for food containers.

Tintometer. Instrument which is used for measuring depth and shade of colour visually by comparison with a range of coloured glass sides. The Lovibond tintometer is the best-known. It is used for the chemical determination of substances that can be converted to coloured compounds, e.g., many minerals and vitamins.

Tisane. French term for a medicinal tea or infusion made from (camomile, lime blossoms, fennel seed, etc).

Tocopherol. Vitamin E.

Tocopheronic Acid. Refers to water-soluble degradation product of alpha-tocopherol (vitamin E) isolated from the urine of animals fed tocopherol, together with tocopheronolactone, the lactone of tocopheronic acid, which is highly vitamin-E active.

Tocopheronic acid is 2-(3-hydroxy-3-methyl-5-carboxyl)-pentyl, 3,5,6-trimethyyl benzoquine.

Toffee. The term used for a sweetmeat that is essentially a dispersion of minute globules of fat in a supersaturated sugar solution. It is made from fat, milk, sugar and confectioners glucose. No real distinction between toffees and caramels except that toffees are boiled at a slightly temperature, 260-270°C compared with 250-255°C for caramels.

Tofu. A Japanese product, soyabean curd. Having 5-8% protein, 3-4% fat, 2-4% carbohydrate and 84-90 % water.

Tomatine. An antifungal substance which is isolated from wiltresistant tomatoes

Tomato. Fruit of Lycopersicon esculentum.

Topfer's Reagent. Dimethylamino-azobenzene; and indicator with a pH range 2.9-40, changing red to yellow. Often used in titration of the acidity of gastric contents, as it changes colour only in the presence of free hydrochloric acid.

Tortilla. Large, flat pancake which is made from ground maize, commonly eaten in Mexico.

Torularhodin. Carotenoid pigment red yeast, Torula, rubra, having vitamin A activity.

Torulin. Antibiotic which is produced during aerobic culture of Torula utilis.

Total Parenteral Nutrition. Dependence entirely on parenteral nutrition.

Tous-les-mois. Queensland arrowroot, used a source or starch.

Toxin. Harmful substances (although many dietary essentials, including some vitamins, have been toxic in large amounts) Generally refer to:

(a) Substance such as cyanide which inhibit metabolic processes;

(b) Those produced by food-poisoning bacteria;

(c) Heavy metals;

(d) A large number of substances occurring in foods which affect nervous system, cause liver damage or are carcinogenic.

TPN.

(1) Abbreviation for triphosphopyridine nucleotide; obsolete name for nicontinamide adenine dinucleotide.

(2) Total parenteral nutrition.

Trace Element. Refers to mineral salts which are needed in small amounts of the order of micrograms milligrams per day-iodine, copper, mangenese, magnesium, zinc, chromium, etc., as distinct from those needed in the hundred milligram range such as calcium, potassium, sodium. Iron is sometimes included as a trace element.

Tragacanth. A gum which is obtained from shrubs of the genus Astragalus. It finds use as emulsifying agent in pharmaceutical preparations and as a thickener.

Transamination. Refers to the transfer of the amino group, $-NH_2$ from one compound to another, usually the influence of an enzyme, transaminase. Thus, glutamic acid under the influence of glutamic-alanine-transaminase conveys its amino group to pyruvic acid to form alanine, leaving keto-glutaric acid.

The prosthetic group of the enzyme is pyridoxal, vitamin B_6, which acts as an intermediate amino carrier.

Transferrin. Or siderophilin. An iron carbonate-protein complex, the form in which iron gets transported in the blood plasma.

Transketolase Test. Enzyme activation Test.

Treacle. First product of refining of molasses from beet sugar cane is black treacle, slightly less bitter; will not crystallise.

Trehalose. Muroom Sugar, also called mycose, a disaccharide : glucopyranosyl-glucopyranoside. It is found in some fungi (Amanita) manna and insects; hydrolysed to glucose.

Tremorgens. Name given to a group of neurotoxins which are produced by various species of moulds (Penicillium, Aspergillus, Claviceps), these cause sustained whole body tremors leading to convulsive seizures which may be fatal (alfatrem from A flavus, penitream from penicillium species). Possible cause of certain endemic afflictions is human beings in Nigeria and India.

Trichinosis (trichiniasis). Disease due to Trichinella spiralis a worm that is a parasite in pork muscle. It is destroyed by heat and by freezing. It is caused by eating undercooked pork or sausage meat.

Trigoneline. Refers to the betaine of nicotinic acid, the form in which nicotinic acid gets excreted in the urine; formula $C_7H_7NO_2$; has no vitamin activity. Also found in seeds of fenugreek and in coffee.

Tri-iodothyronine. Refers to the active hormone of the

thyroid gland into which thyroxine is converted in the tissues. It is synthesised in the body from the acid tyrosine and iodine.

Triotin. Unidentified urinary excretion product of biotin, together within miotin and rhiotin.

Tripe. Refers to the lining of the stomach of ruminants, usually calf or ox. According to the part of stomach used, there are various kinds like blanket, honeycomb, book, monk's hood and reed tripe. It is having large amounts of connective tissue which gets converted into gelatin on boiling; sold 'dressed' i.e., cleaned and treated with lime.

Triticale. Cross between wheat (Triticum) and rye (Secale) which combines the winter harliness of the rye with the special properties of wheat.

Truffle. Edible fungus that grows underground and is detected by trained dogs or pigs.

Trypsin. Proteolytic enzyme of the pancreatic juice which attacks parts of the protein molecule left unattacked by pepsin. It functions at alkaline pH, 8-11. Secreted as the inactive precursor, trypsinogen; liberated by enterokinse.

Tryptophan. Amino indole propionic acid. It is an essential amino acid. It gets destroyed by acid; therefore protein analysis requires a separate alkaline hydrolysis.

Tuberin. Refers to potato, a globulin.

Tuber. Underground storage organ of some plants, e.g, potato Jerusalem artichoke, sweet potato, yam.

Tun. A vat having 210 imperial gallons.

Tuna. Or tunny. Fatty fish, species of Thunnus and Neothunnus. Also name for prickly pear.

Turmeric. Dried rhizome of Curcuma longa (ginger family), grown in India and S. Asia. Deep yellow and used both as condiment and (permitted) dyestuff. Used is curry powder and in prepared mustard. Its pigment is used as a dye under the name curcumin.

Turnip. Root of Brassica campestris.

Tyramine. 4-Hydroxyphenethylamine. It is also called

tyrosamine, which is formed by decarboxylation of the amino acid tyrosine. Found in ripened cheese; stimulates the sympathetic system and can cause increased blood pressure and may be cause of migraine.

Normally destroyed by monoamine oxidases, but certain drugs inhibit these enzymes and patients on such drugs must avoid cheese and other foods which contain similar amines, including wine, chocolate and yeast preparations.

Tyrosinase. An enzyme that is able to oxidise tyrosine and other phenolic compounds, with the ultimate production of brown and black pigments. Absent in albinos, and from the white areas of piebald animals.

It occurs in the potato and is responsible for the dark colour produced when raw potatoes or the juice are allowed to autoxidise in air.

Tyrosine. Non-essential amino acid that is having some sparing action on the essential amino acid phenylalanine. It is very little soluble and crystallises out of solutions of protein hydrolysates.

Tyrosine is the starting material for the formation of melanin the pigment in the hair skin, increased after sunburn. Chemically it is amino hydroxyphenyl propionic acid.

Tyrosinosis. Refers to an inborn error of metabolism in which there occurs failure of enzyme p-hydroxyphenylpyruvate hydroxlase, so that the normal metabolic path of tyrosine to homogentisic acid cannot be followed and tyrosine, hydroxyphenylpyruvate, lactate and acetate get excreted in the urine. The defect appears to be harmless.

reptiles and of purine metabolism in man and the anthropoid apes. Other mammal are having the enzyme uricase, which converts the uric acid to allantoin.

Uricotelic. Animals that excrete their waste nitrogen as uric acid, e.g. birds and reptiles.

Urobilinogen. Pigment in urine which is derived from the bile pigments, which, in turn, are formed from haemoglobin. When urine is left to stand, the urobilinogen is oxidised in air to urobilin.

Urogastrone. A hormone similar to gastrin found in urine; little known of its function.

Uropepsin. Proteolytic enzyme in urine. It is produced by acidification of uropepsinogen, which is identical with gastric pepsinogen. Urinary output serves as a measure of the amount of peptic glandular tissues.

V

Vacuum Contact Plate Process. Refers to the method of dehydrating food in a vacuum oven in which material is heated by not plates both above and below. As the material shrinks owing to water losses, continuous contact is maintained by closing of the plates. Has the advantage over a simple vacuum oven of supplying heat more effectively to the food. Also known as VCD–vacuum contact dryer.

Valine. An essential amino acid, rarely, if ever, limiting in foods. Chemically, amino isovaleric acid.

Vanadium. Element which is not shown to be essential but found in several animal tissues, and believed to play a biological role.

Vanaspati. Purified, hydrogenated, vegetable oil. It is used in India and similar to margarine; fortified with vitamin A and vitamin D.

Vanilla. Refers to the extract of the vanilla bean, fruit of the orchid Aracus aromatics (or Vanilla aromaticus) and related species. Fruits area allowed to formet, when the beans become dark brown in colour; they are crushed and extracted with alcohol.

Chief flavouring principle has been vanillin or methyl protacatechuic aldehyde, but other substances present aid the flavour, and synthetic vanillin has not the true flavour.

Vanilla sugar–ground bean mixed with sugar.

Ethyl vanillin–a synthetic substance, does not occur in the vanilla bean; incorrectly named–ethyl replaces methyl of vanillin; 3½ times strong in flavour, and more stable to storage than vanillin.

Vasoconstriction. Constriction of the blood vessel; the reserve of vasodilation.

Vasodilation. Refers to Dilation of the blood vessels; the reverse is vasoconstriction. Caused by a rise in body temperature and serves to lose heat from the body.

Veal. Most of the young calf, not less than 3 weeks old.

Vegans. Refers to these who consume to animal foods. (Vegetarians often consume milk and /or eggs).

Vegetables Butters. Refers to the naturally occurring fats that melt rather sharply because they are having a preponderance of a single triglyceride.

Cocoa butter–from Theobroma cacoa bean, used in chocolate; Borneo tallow or green butter–from Malayam and East Indian plant, Shorea, stenoptera, resembles cocoa butter; shea butter– from African plant, Butyro spermum parkii, softer than cocoa butter. Mowrah fat or illipe butter–from Indian plant, Bassia longifolia, used for soap and candles.

Vegetable Protein Products. General term to include textured soya products which are often made to simulate meat. Basic material is called flour when the protein content is not less than 50%; concentrate, not less than 65%; isolate, not than 90%; protein.

Vegetables. Refers to the plant or parts of plants which are cultivated for food. Some foods that are botanically fruits, such as tomatoes and cucumbers, and seeds, like peas and beans, are included with the vegetables.

As a source of nutrients most of the vegetables are useful sources of vitamin C and minerals, the root vegetables supply carbohydrate, but only the seeds are an important sources of protein.

Verbascose. Refers to a tetrasaccharide, galactose-galactose- glucose-fructose which is found in legumes. It passes down the intestine (along with raffinose and stachyose), where it gets fermented by bacteria and causes flatulence.

Verjuice. Originally the juice of carb apples, now lemon juice used in cooking meat or fish.

Vermouth. The term used for the wine to which has been added a mixture of aromatic and bitter herbs, such as angelica, cinchona, coriander, wormwood, angostura, etc.

Vicilin. Globulin protein which occurs in pea and lentil.

Vienna Bread. Loaf having a very crisp, thin, highly glazed crust, with cuts on the upper surface, coarser than ordinary bread and with gas holes. It gets baked in an oven which retains the steam.

Vieth's Ratio. With reference to milk is the ratio anhydrous lactose : protein : ash, which is normally 13 : 9 : 2.

Villi, Intestinal. Refers to the small, finger-like processes which are covering the surfaces of the small intestine in large numbers. They provide and enormous surface area for the absorption of digested food from the small intestine.

Vinasses. Refers to the residual liquors from sugar-beet molasses. They contain appreciable quantities of betaine.

Vinegar. Refers to the product of a double fermentation, first to ethanol then to acetic acid, effected by Acetobacter. The film of Acetobacter on the surface of the liquid is known as 'mother of vinegar '.

It is having about 5% acetic acid, with flavours derived from esters and higher alcohols; often referred to as wine, malt or cider vinegar, as distinct from a 5% solution of acetic acid–sometimes called 'non-brewed vinegar'.

Viosterol. Irradiated ergosterol *i.e.*, vitamin D_2.

Viscogen. Thickening agent for whipping cream. Two parts of lime (CaO) in six parts of water, added to five parts of sugar in ten parts of water; used at the rate of $\frac{1}{2}$– oz per gallon of cream.

Viscometer. An instrument which is used for measuring the viscosity of liquids.

Viscosity. Team used of liquids to define their resistance to flow (*i.e.* the internal friction).

Visual Purple (rhodopsin). A pigment which is present in the retina of the eye, and consisting of retinol plus protein, which is necessary for vision in dim light.

Vitamers. Substances structurally related to vitamins, having some biological activity, though often less than the pure vitamin.

Vitamin. Refers to a naturally occurring organic substance which is essential in very small amounts for the normal functioning of the living cell. Hence a factor essential for an animal or micro-organisms and not essential for man is, nevertheless, called a vitamin.

It is now questionable whether it is desirable to group together substances as varied in function as, for example, the B vitamins, which function as coenzymes, and substances like vitamin D, which appears to function as a hormone.

Vitamin A. Includes both retinol (previously called preformed vitamin A) and carotene (previously termed vitamin A precursor). It is essential for formation of glycoproteins of the mucous tissue by acting as a carrier for the monosaccharides, involved; thus, maintains normal condition of moist epithelial tissues lining mouth, respiratory and urinary tract; essential for growth. The aldehyde, retinal, is required for vision in dim light in combination with protein to form visual purple.

Deficiency given use to night blindness, xerophthalmia (drying of tear ducts) and keratomalacia (ulceration of the cornea), blindness and stunting of growth. It occurs as in fish liver oils (cod and halibut), milk and butter, and as carotene in green vegetable, carrots and palm oil.

Daily recommended in take 750µ for adult (2500 i.u.). Vitamin A content of foods expressed as retinol equivalents; 1µg retinol = 6µg beta-carotene = 12µ other active carotenoids = 3.3 i.u. retinol = 0 i.u. beta-carotene.

Vitamin A_2. Old name for dehydroretinol, the form which is found in livers of freshwater fish; has 40% of biological activity of retinol.

Vitamin B Complex. See under individual B vitamins. These vitamins all found together in cereal germ, liver and yeast; are all coenzymes; and historically were discovered by separation from what was known originally as 'vitamin B' : hence, they are grouped together as the B complex. The vitamin B_2 complex is of purely historical origin and includes all except B_1.

Vitamin B_c. Folic acid.

Vitamin B_p. Called the antiperosis factor for chicks, but can gets replaced by manganese and choline.

Vitamin B_T. Refers to an essential dietary factor for the mealworm. Tenebrio molitor, and certain related species; now known to be identical with carnitine. In higher animals carnitine plays a part in fat synthesis by transferring acetyl across the mitochondrial membrane but it is not a dietary essential.

Vitamin B_w. Or factor W. It is probably identical with biotin.

Vitamin B_x. Non-existent : has been used in the past for both pantothenic acid and para-amino benzoic acid.

Vitamin B_1. Thiamin. Thiamin pyrophosphate is the coenzyme, cocarboxylase which is required in oxidative decarboxylation, e.g. the conversion of ketogtarate to succinate and of pyruvic acid to acetyl. A deficiency of the vitamin give rise impair metabolism of carbohydrate and clinically results in the disease berriberri, in which pyruvate accumulates in the blood.

The daily requirement is related to the amount of carbohydrate oxidized (the non-fat calories)–0.6mg per 1000 non-fat calories or 0.4mg per 1000 total calories (daily total approximately 1mg). Thiamin is water-soluble and there occurs little storage in the body.

It is found in cereal grains (little in white flour and white rise but these are enriched with added thiamin in many countries), in yeast, meat, especially pork, pluses, egg.

It has been one of the more labile of the vitamins and gets destroyed by heat under alkaline conditions and by sulphur dioxide, and gets lost by leaching into the cooking water. The baking of bread can give rise to 15-30% loss; up to half can be lost in cooked meat and fish, depending on the conditions.

Vitamin B_2. Riboflavin. In combination with many different proteins it forms a group of coenzymes called flavoproteins, essential for the oxidation of carbohydrates. Flavoproteins act as intermediary hydrogen carriers and include flavin mono-nucleotide, flavin adenine dinucleotide, cytochrome creductase, etc. A deficiency of riboflavin impairs cell oxidation and results clinically in a set of symptoms called ariboflavinosis. These include cracking of the skin at the corners of the mouth (angular stomatitis), fissuring of the lips (cheilosis) and tongue changes (glossitis); seborrhoeic accumulations appear around the nose and eyes.

Recommended intake is about 0.55 mg per 100 kcal or an average of 1.5mg per day. It is found in yeast, liver, milk, eggs, cheese and pulses.

Processing losses occur partly due to leaching into the water and partly to exposure to light 50% of the riboflavin of milk can get destroyed in 2 hours by exposure to bright sunlight, and even on a dull day the losses can be 20%. The products of photoxidation of the vitamin B_2 destroy the vitamin C.

Vitamin B_3. Non-existent ; term which was once used for pantothenic acid and sometimes ; quite wrongly, used for niacin.

Vitamin B_4. Name assigned to what was later identified as a mixture of arginine, glycine and cystine.

Vitamin B_5. Name assigned to a substance which was later presumed to be identical with vitamin B_6 or possibly nicotinic acid.

Vitamin B_6. Generic descriptor for three derivatives of 2-methyl-pyridine, namely the hydroxy compound, pyridoxine (previously known as adermin and pyridoxol), the aldehyde, pyridoxal, and the amine, pyridoxamine; all equally active.

Deficiency brings about convulsions and acrodynia (skin disorder) in rats, abnormal red cells in dairy cattle, anaemia in dogs and epileptiform seizures in human babies.

It functions as coenzyme for specific amino acid decarboxylases and deaminases, transminases and transmethylases.

It is rarely deficient in human diets. It recommended intake is thought to be about 2 mg per day. It is found in nuts, meat, fish, whole grain.

Vitamin B_7. When a new factor was discovered which was claimed to be essential for chick growth and feathering, the claimant stated that as nine factors were known the new factors should be termed as vitamins B_{10} and B_{11}. In fact, the B vitamins had been numbered only up to B_6, hence B_7, B_8 and B_9 have never existed.

Vitamin B_8. Vitamin B_7.

Vitamin B_9. Vitamin B_7.

Vitamin B_{10}. The names B_{10} and B_{11} were assigned to two factors claimed to be essential or chick growth and feathering; they were later shown to be a mixture of vitamin B_1 and folic acid.

Vitamin B_{11}. Vitamin B_{10}.

Vitamin B_{12}. Generic descriptor for the cobalamins. They are water-soluble organic compounds consisting of a corrin nucleus of four linked pyrrole rings linked to a cobalt atom. Hydroxocobalamin (formerly B_{12a}) and aquocobalamin (B_{12}b) are the active forms; cyanocobalamin occurs in small amounts in blood plasma but dies not have an active role.

It is essential for nucleic acid synthesis and so for formation of red blood cells. Pernicious anaemia occurs due to inability to absorb the B_{12} because of lack of factor in the stomach termed the intrinsic factor, rather than a dietary deficiency of the vitamin (formerly called the extrinsic factor).

Vitamin B_{13}. It is not an established vitamin.

Vitamin B_{14}. Not an established vitamin; a substance which occurs in human urine which gets increased the rate of cell-proliferation in bone-marrow culture.

Vitamin B_{15}. Pangamic acid, which see; no evidence that it is a dietary essential.

Vitamin B_{16}. This term has never been used.

Vitamin C. L-xylo-ascobic acid (the isomer, D-araboascorbic acid, or isoascorbic acid or erythorbic acid, is having only slight biological activity, 1/20th, but finds use as an antioxidant in foods. It controls production of intercellular cementing substances, because it is essential for the hydroxylation of praline to hydroxyproline, a step in the synthesis of collagen. Breakdown of this matrix allow seepage of blood from capillaries, subcutaneous bleeding, weakness of muscles, soft, spongy gums leading to loss teeth—in other words, scurvy. It is readily oxidised, especially in foods kept hot, and leached into cooking water.

It is found in fruits and vegetables; used as antioxidant and bread improver.

D-xyloascorbic acid, L-araboascorbic and having zero biological activity; L-rhamno-has 1/5th of activity of vitamin C; D-arabo-has 1/20th.

Vitamin D. Produced in the skin under the action of ultraviolet light which converted 7-dehydrocholesterol into vitamin D_5 or cholecalciferol. It is also synthesised as vitamin D_2 or ergocalciferol by irradiation of ergosterol.

Term vitamin D_1 was assigned originally to an impure mixture and is not used now.

It gets converted into 25-hydroxy derivative in liver and then into 1,25-dihydroxy derivative in kidney. This 10 times more potent than vitamin D and stimulates absorption of dietary calcium from intestine and calcium turnover in bone.

Deficiency brings about rickets in young children, osteomalacia in adults. Not widely distributed in foods–egg yolk, butter, fatty fish and enriched margarine Recommended intakes 10μg (400 i.u.) for infants and children 2.5 μg (100 i.u.) for adults. Excess can be harmful.

Vitamin E. Generic term for group of fat-soluble compounds which are essential for reproduction in animals. Essential for man (not for reproduction, so far as is known) but rarely, if ever, deficient animal species—sterility in mouse, rat, rabbit, sheep and turkey; muscular dystrophy in several species; capillary permeability in chick and turkey; anaemian in monkey. Many substances are having vitamin E—like activity, eight in particular (old names in parentheses) : 5, 7, 8-trimethyl tocotrienol (alpha-tocotrienol) (gamma); and 8- mythyltocotrienol (delta). All expressed as alpha-tocopherol equivalents.

These compounds are antioxidants with varying potencies, and their natural occurrence in vegetable oils is able to protect the latter against rancidity.

Vitamin F. Essential fatty acids.

Vitamin G. D obsolete name for vitamin B_2.

Vitamin H. Biotin.

Vitamin K. Fat-soluble vitamin which is essential for the production by the liver of prothrombin and several others factors involved in the bloods clotting system. Hence, it is called the antihaemorrhagic vitamin.

It is widely distributed in greenstuffs and synthesised by bacteria in the intestine but not known how much gets absorbed; dietary deficiency is not encountered (except in newborn infants with a sterile intestine) only failure of absorption.

Vitamin L. Vitamin L_1 and L_2 are factors in yeast which are said to be essential for lactation; they have not become established.

Vitaminoids. Name assigned to compounds with 'vitamin-like', activity, that is, considered by some to be vitamins or partially to replace vitamins-include bioflavonoids (formerly vitamin P), mesoinositol, carnitine, choline, lipoic acid and the essential fatty acid (formerly vitamin F).

Vitamin P. Name formerly assigned to a group of plant flavonoid substances which affect the strength of the walls of the blood capillaries—namely, rutin (buckwheat), hesperiden. Eriodiction and citrin (in the pith of citrus fruits). (Citrin is a mixture of hesperidin and eriopictin). Now believed that the effect is pharmacological and that they are not dietary essential; sometimes called 'bioflavonoids'. It is called vitamin P from 'phameabilitats vitamins'. Once claimed as a crue for the common cold.

Vitamin T. ρ factor which occurs in insect cuticle, mould mycelia and yeast fermentation liquor, claimed to accerlerate maturation and promoteprotein synthesis. Also called torulitine. Said to be a mixture of folic acid, vitamin B_{12} and desoxyribosides and not a new factor.

Vitellin. One of the proteins of egg yolk. It is approximately four-fifths of the total protein. It is a phosphorus of egg yolf.

VLDL. Very low-density lipoproteins.

Vodka. Made from neutral spirit, *i.e.* alcohol distillate (in Russia mainly from potatoes), with little or no acid present, so that there occurs no ester formation and, hence, no flavour.

Vol. Trade name which is used for commercial ammonium carbonate, a mixture of ammonium bicarbonate and carbamate. It is used as aerating agent. In baking, as it breaks down when heated to give carbon dioxide, ammonia and steam, without leaving any residue.

Votator. Machine which is used for the continuous manufacture of margarine; the fact and water get emulsified, and the subsequent conditioning process carried out in the same machine.

W

Warburg's Yellow Enzyme. Refers to a flavoprotein that is part of the cell oxidation chain; passes on the hydrogen from reduced coenzyme 1 to cytochrome.

Water, Demineralised. Refers to water that has been purified by passage through a bed of ion-exchange resin which removes minerals salts. Demineralised or deionised water is as pure as, and can be purer than, distilled water.

Water Hardness. Refers to soap-precipitating power of water because of the formation of insoluble calcium and magnesium salts of the soap. Temporary hardness can be removed by boiling, permanent hardness is not. May be measured in degree Clerke; one degree = 1 part of calcium carbonate per 1000000 parts of water.

Water-soluble Vitamins. Refers to all the members of the B. Complex (thiamin, riboflavin, nicotinic acid, pantothenic acid, pyridoxine, biotin, folic acid, para-amino benzonic acid, choline, inositol and vitamin B_{12}) and vitamin C. Unlike the storage of vitamins A and D in the liver, there occurs no specific site for storage of the water-soluble vitamins; they are merely dispersed in solution through the blood and tissues.

Waxes. Esters of fatty acids having long-chain monohydric alcohols (fats are esters of fatty acids with the three-carbon trihydric alcohol, glycerol). For example, beeswax, ester of palmitic acid with myricyl alcohol; spermaceti, cetyl palmitate. Animal waxes are often esters of the steroid alcohol, cholesterol.

Weende Analysis. Refers to analysis of foods and feedingstuffs for nitrogen, either extract, crude fibre and ash together with soluble carbohydrate calculated by subtracting these values from the total.

Weight-for-age. Standard weight-for-age refers to the 50th centile of the weight-for-age curves of well-fed children.

Weighting Oils. Brominated oils.

Wetzel Grid. Children have been grouped by physique into five groups, ranging from tall and thin to short and thick-set. A healthy child will grow, as measured by height and weight, along one of these channels at a standard rate, if he deviates from the channel malnutrition is suspected.

Wey. 48 bushels of oats or 40 bushels of salt or 'corn'.

Whalemeat. Analysis per 100g (edible portion only); protein 20g, fat 4g, kcal 125 (0.53MJ), Fe 2.4mg vitamin B_1 0.03mg, vitamin B_2 0.1mg, nicotinic acid 4.4mg.

Whale Oil. Used, after hardening by hydrogenation, for lower quality margarines, also in soap making.

Whey. Refers to the residue from milk after removal of the casein and most of the fat (as in cheese-making); also known as lactoserum.

Having about 1% protein (lactalbumin and lactoglobulin) together with all lactose, water-soluble vitamins and minerals, and therefore has some food value, although it is 92% water. Whey cheese can be made by heat coagulation of the protein, and whey butter from the small amount (0.25%) fat.

Dried whey is added to processed cheese; most whey is fed in liquid form to pigs.

Whey Butter. Butter, Whey.

Whiskey, whisky. A grain spirit which is distilled from barley, rye or other cereal which has first been malted and then fermented. Most brands of whisky are a blend of pure malt whisky with spirit distilled from grain.

White Blood Cells. Leucocytes.

White Cell Count. Leucocytes.

White Rice. Rice.

Whole-wheat Meal. Flour or meal which is prepared by milling the whole wheat grain, i.e., 100% extraction rate.

Wills' Factor. A factor in autolysed yeast which is effective in promoting red blood cell formation, probably folic acid.

Wine. Fermented grape juice having 9-10% w/v ethyl alcohol. Beverages made by fermenting other fruit juices and sugar in the presence of vegetables or leaves or roots are also called wines (parsnip, peapod, oak leaf wine, etc.), although the legal definition may be restricted to the fermented grape.

Wineberry. Rubus phoenicolasius. It is similar to rasberry, orange coloured.

Winterisation. Applied to edible oils, which means the removal of the more saturated glycerides of that the oil remains bright and clear at low temperatures. The oil is simply chilled and the solidified palmitates and stearates filtered off.

Witches Milk. Refers to the secretion of the mammary gland of the newborn of both sexes, due to the presence of the hormone prolactin that travels from the blood of the mother into the fetus. Also known as sorceres' milk.

Wood Alcohol. Methyl alcohol CH_3OH; highly toxic. Its presence in methylated spirits accounts for the toxicity of the latter.

Worcester Sauce. Characterised by spicy flavour, sediment and thin supernatant liquid. Recipes usually secret but basically soya, tamarinds, anchovies, garlic and spices, plus sugar, salt and vinegar, matured 6 months in oak casks.

World Food Programme. The part of Food and Agriculture Organization of the United Nations which is intended to give international aid in the form of food countries with a surplus.

X

Xanthine Oxidase. Refers to an enzyme which is present in milk and in liver, specific for the two purines xanthine and hypoxanthine (which is oxidises to uric acid), and will also oxidise a range of aldehydes to the corresponding acids. It is identical with Scharodinger's enzyme of milk.

Xanthophylls. The collective term for hydroxylated carotenoids or carotenols.

Xanthoproteic Test. For proteins (actually for the benzene nucleus of tyrosine and tryptophan which occur in nearly all proteins). Yellow colour on boiling with nitric acid, turns orange on adding ammonia.

Xenobiotic. Substances foreign to the body, including drugs and some food additives.

Xerophthalmia. Found in advanced vitamin A deficiency. Epithelium of the cornea and conjunctiva of the eye deteriorates due to impairment of the tear glands, causing dryness then ulceration.

Xylitol. Five-carbon sugar alcohol which is corresponding to the sugar xylulose. As sweet as sucrose, less prone to cause dental decay and used in some; sugar free products like chewing gum.

Xylose. Pentose sugar occurring in plant tissues as complex polysaccharide; 40% sweetness of sucrose.

Xylulose. Five-carbon sugar-alcohol which is derived from the pentose sugar xyloxe.

Y

Yeast Fermentation, Bottom. Refers to fermentation during the manufacturing of beer with a yeast that sinks to the bottom of the bank. Most beers are produced this way; ale, porter and stout being the principal beers produced by top fermentation.

Yeast. Grouped with the fungi although they are unicellular. Various types are of major importance in the food industry.

Yellow Colours. Oil Yellow GG-mixture of 4-phenylazoresorcinol and 4,6-di- (phenylazo) resorcinol.

Sunset yellow FCF-disodium salt of 1-p-sulphophenylazo-2-naphthol-6-sulphonic acid; yellow-orange colour used to simulate the colour of eggs or orange; called Yellow No. 6 in the USA.

Yoghurt. Milks, fermented.

Yolk Index. Index of freshness of an egg. Refers to the ratio between height and diameter of yolk defined conditions. As the egg deteriorates, the yolk index gets decreased.

Yuksov Disease. Another name for Haff disease.

Z

Zest. Outer skin of citrus fruits.

Zinc. Refers to a dietary essential that is part of the structure of about 20 enzymes, including carbonic anhydrase, alcohol dehydrogenase and superoxide dismutase.

Zomotherap. Treatment of convalescents with raw meat or juice-long since discontinued.

Zoopherin. Vitamin B_{12}.

Zooplankton. Wide variety of very small crustaceans and other invertebrates which are mixed with the young of larger fish, which live upon the phytoplankton (although some are carnivorous) and serve, in turn, as a food supply of small fish and other marine life.

Zwieback. German term for twice-baked bread. It is ordinary dough plus eggs and butter, baked, sliced, baked again to a rusk and sometimes sugar coated.

Zymase. Name assigned to the mixture of enzymes in yeast which is responsible for fermentation.

Zymogens. Refer to the inactive form in which some enzymes exist before being liberated by the action of a kinase. For example, trypsinogen and pepsinogen are secreted in the intestine and converted into their active forms, trypsin and pepsin.

Zymotachygraph. Refers to an instrument that is able to measure the gas produced in a fermenting dough and the amount escaping from the dough.

❑❑❑